CNA Study Guide 2024-2025

Review Book with 300 Practice Questions & Answer Explanations for the Certified Nursing Assistant Exam

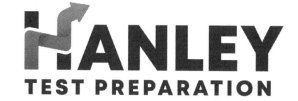

HANLEY
TEST PREPARATION

Contents

Free Video Offer!

Thank you for purchasing from Hanley Test Preparation! We're honored to help you prepare for your exam. To show our appreciation, we're offering an Exclusive Test Tips Video.

This video includes multiple strategies that will make you successful on your big exam.

All we ask is that you email us your feedback and describe your experience with our product. Amazing, awful, or just so-so. We want to hear what you have to say!

To get your FREE VIDEO, just send us an email at bonusvideo@hanleytestprep.com with **Free Video** in the subject line and the following information in the body of the email:

- The name of the product you purchased
- Your product rating on a scale of 1-5, with 5 being the highest rating.
- Your feedback about the product.

If you have any questions or concerns, please don't hesitate to contact us at support@hanleytestprep.com

Thanks again!

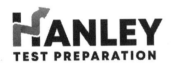

Introduction

In your early twenties, you are at a pivotal point in your life. What should be your career path? Let's say you are vying for the healthcare profession. Many of your acquaintances are in the healthcare industry, and how they draw attention and enjoy social status has made you lean toward this profession as an immediate career choice. Additionally, post-Covid, the world is reeling from job crunches and loss. A career in health care, however, is one that is flourishing and in high demand. It has a variety of positions that pay much over the median wage in the country.

Significantly, the contemporary healthcare scenario in the US affirms your decision to enter into the sector. According to the US Census Bureau's projections, the United States' population is leaning toward an aging demography. Currently, 1 in 6 Americans are 65 or older, increasing healthcare demands (Caplan, 2023). Moreover, quality healthcare is facing a critical shortage of nurses and other nursing staff (Hilgers, 2023). The LinkedIn data shares the high demand for nursing personnel in the expanding healthcare industry.

Since Florence Nightingale elevated nursing to a noble profession, many women have found success in this field. There are only a few professions where a woman's nurturing and caring qualities are equally valued and compensated for. Whether it is the ultimate goal, it is always discerning and pragmatic to be open to opportunities to expand your network, education, and work history. Starting as a nursing assistant is the most fantastic way to gain field experience. It's an opportunity to familiarize yourself with the nursing profession while earning.

Nursing assistants must finish a state-approved curriculum at high schools, community colleges, vocational and technical institutions, hospitals, and nursing homes. A brief on-the-job training is required to learn an employer's regulations and processes. Clearing the competence exam grants a state-specific license or certification for registry enrollment.

Some states designate nursing assistants as certified nursing assistants (CNA). States might mandate continued education and a criminal background verification by certifying authorities. Some states provide scope for additional credentials like Certified Medical Assistant (CMA) who can dispense medications (Nursing Assistants and Orderlies, 2023).

CNA programs can be excellent "starter careers" or ways to promote further schooling in healthcare. High school CNA programs can have better examination pass rates than third-party programs, making it a viable career option for high school students (An Overview of CNA Shortage, 2023).

The certified nursing assistant examination comprises a written or oral test and a clinical skills test. A third-party test appointee takes the written part of the test. The two-part multiple-choice question type of test format typically needs two hours to complete. It has questions from anatomy, physiology, and other subjects, including medical terminology. You must know CNA roles and responsibilities. A nurse or other practitioner conducts a clinical skills examination. Clinical tests require knowledge of practices of hand-washing, pulse checking, measuring blood pressure, and other miscellaneous skills from a list of over 20. Passing scores for CNA tests vary according to the state and can range from 70%–80%.

You can take the test three times within two years of completing the training program. Retesting requires clearing only those sections that you failed.

CNA certification is typically valid for two years. Renewal is straightforward if you continue working for designated hours as a CNA during this term (with statewide variation). Not satisfying the renewal criteria and license expiry for two years or less can mandate a competence test for renewal by some states. Enrolling in the CNA program to apply for a fresh CNA license is mandatory if it has expired for an extended period or is ineligible for renewal.

How do you crack the CNA test? How best to navigate unknown medical terms and phrases or learn to record blood pressure correctly? Before giving up or declaring that it is impossible, pause and relax. You have found this book. You no longer have to keep your dream a secret. This book will tell you what to do concisely and accurately.

Nurses in Northern Ireland launched a regional program known as the PACE (Person-centered Assessment, Care Planning, and Evaluation) Framework to raise the bar on care planning. The 'PACE' Framework results from an iterative process. PACE for nursing care planning has contributed to the growth of person-centered practice.

This guidebook underscores the importance of PACE to shift from task orientation care toward person-centered care. PACE helps you to identify areas of action and how to appraise them. The process gives you confidence and a solid foundation in the subject.

The book functions as a catalyst in initiating an action, in this case, strategic examination preparation and accomplishment. To your surprise, you will find that you no longer need to memorize things. They are archived in your brain automatically through the carefully designed study path. The skills you learn can eventually help you to elevate to the rank of a registered nurse (RN).

Nursing requires communication, compassion, patience, and endurance. If you have these excellent qualities, look no further to establish a nursing career with the help of this guidebook.

In time, you will succeed as the best professional and be a mentor to new learners.

Part One: Examination Content Review

Chapter One: CNA Examination Overview

This chapter discusses the CNA examination in detail to help you understand what it means to be a nursing assistant and how best to approach the test. For instance, what is the most critical step in approaching a competitive examination? Licensing tests allow you to practice a particular field of study. Hence, knowing about that *field* and the *test* itself is vital to succeeding with high scores.

It means the world of tests is not fraught with constant study and cramming of materials. What you learn today, you can forget tomorrow. It raises frustration and stress. When unchecked, stress can even lead to examination phobia, offsetting the primary purpose of the examination, *caring for one's health*. Exploring the structure of the CNA test will help us know our challenger. We will learn about the aim and direction of the test to gain test aptitude.

CNA Examination

The National Association of Health Care Assistants describes the CNA's role as healthcare workers in a nursing home or hospital setting who help older adults with everyday living tasks and chronically ill or rehabilitation patients unable to self-care.

Requirements for CNA certification vary among states. They include the following:

- Accredited CNA program.
- Pass the state's CNA test with written and practical aspects.
- State registration as CNA.
- Perform a minimum number of hours of supervised duty as a nursing assistant.

States, Registration, Eligibility, and Test Administration

The following states accept CNA certification with statewide variation in requirements and modes of examination:

- Alabama

    o State-approved CNA program (75 hours, including 16 hours of clinical and 16 hours of lab)
    o Nurse Aide Certification by Examination through Pearson VUE or Prometric

- Alaska

    o State-approved CNA program (140 hours, including 60 hours of classroom instruction and 80 hours of clinics or lab)
    o Nurse Aide Certification by Examination through Pearson VUE.

- Arizona

    o Board-approved CNA program (minimum 120 hours of training)
    o State written and manual aptitude exam through HDmaster
    o Legal residency proof

- Arkansas

- o State-approved CNA program (minimum 90 hours)
- o Nursing Assistant Competency Exam through Prometric

- California

  - o Minimum 16 years old.
  - o Authorized CNA training program.
  - o Criminal record clearance.
  - o Competency Evaluation Examination

- Colorado

  - o State-sanctioned CNA training program
  - o NNAAP through Pearson VUE

- Connecticut

  - o Board-approved CNA program (apply for certification within 24 months of completion)
  - o Connecticut Nurse Aide examination by Prometric

- Delaware

  - o State-sanctioned training program
  - o CNA competency test through Prometric

- Florida

  - o Approved CNA training program (a student may plan to apply for certification by test only)
  - o A minimum score on the nursing assistant competency examination through Prometric

- Georgia

  - o Board-sanctioned CNA program
  - o Qualify NNAAP through Pearson VUE

- Hawaii

  - o State-approved CNA training program
  - o Hawaii Nurse Aide Competency Exam administered through Prometric

- Idaho

  - o State-sanctioned training program (120 hours)
  - o Idaho Nurse Aide Exam through Prometric

- Illinois

  - o Illinois-sanctioned training course
  - o Written test

- Indiana

  - o Nurse Aide Training Program (105 hours)
  - o Written and skills test

- Iowa

  - o Approved CNA course (75 hours)
  - o Written and skills test

- Kansas

  - o Approved CNA training program (90 hours)
  - o State CNA examination with a 75% score or more

- Kentucky

  - o Approved CNA course (at least 75 hours with 16 hours of supervised clinical training)
  - o Final examination (written or oral and skills test)
  - o Competency evaluation

- Louisiana

    o   State-approved CNA training program
    o   CNA certification test

- Maine

    o   State-approved CNA program (180 hours of training)
    o   Maine CNA competency test
    o   Criminal background check

- Maryland

    o   Board-approved CNA program (100 hours of instruction)
    o   CNA competency test (written and manual aptitudes)

- Massachusetts

    o   Department-sanctioned Nurse Aide Training Program
    o   Nurse Aide Competency Evaluation test (four attempts for passing the knowledge portion and three for clinical)

- Michigan

    o   State nursing assistant program
    o   Evaluation test by Prometric with a 2-year certification

- Minnesota

    o   State-approved CNA training program
    o   Competency evaluation test

    Or,

    o   Excellent status on a nursing assistant registration in another state with 8 hours of CNA job in the previous 24 months

- Mississippi

  - o Completion of approved CNA program
  - o NNAAP by Pearson VUE

- Missouri

  - o State-approved CNA training program (75 hours classroom theory and 100 hours on-job)
  - o State CNA certification test

- Montana

  - o State-approved CNA training program
  - o State CNA certification test through HDmaster

- Nebraska

  - o Age at least 16 years old
  - o Minimum 75 hours of state-approved training or a 21-hour introductory resident-care class for intermediate care facilities for individuals with developmental disabilities.
  - o One-hour Nebraska-specific abuse or neglect or misappropriation training
  - o Nebraska-approved written or oral and skills competency tests

- Nevada

  - o State-sanctioned Nurse Aide Training Program
  - o State CNA test through HDmaster

- New Hampshire

  - o State-sanctioned Nurse Aide Training Program
  - o State CNA test through HDmaster

- New Jersey

- o State-sanctioned Nurse Aide Training Program
- o State CNA test through HDmaster

- New Mexico

  - o State-sanctioned Nurse Aide Training Program
  - o State CNA test through Prometric

- New York

  - o State-sanctioned Nurse Aide Training Program
  - o State CNA test through Prometric

- North Carolina

  - o State-sanctioned nurse-aide training program (75 hours or more)
  - o State CNA test through Pearson VUE

- North Dakota

  - o State-sanctioned Nurse Aide Training Program
  - o State CNA test through HDmaster

- Ohio

  - o State-sanctioned Nurse Aide Training Program
  - o State CNA test through HDmaster

- Oklahoma

  - o State-sanctioned Nurse Aide Training Program
  - o State CNA test through HDmaster

- Oregon

  - o State-sanctioned Nurse Aide Training Program
  - o Criminal background check
  - o Competency test by Hdmaster

- Pennsylvania

  - o State-sanctioned Nurse Aide Training Program
  - o Competency test by Credential within 24 months of the program's ending

- Rhode Island

  - o State-approved CNA training program (120 hours of training)
  - o Application for a nursing assistant license
  - o CNA competency test

- South Carolina

  - o State-sanctioned CNA training program.
  - o SC Nurse Aide exam through Pearson VUE

- South Dakota

  - o Training program authorized by the SD Board of Nursing
  - o Competency test through HDmaster
  - o Minimum 16 years of age

- Tennessee

  - o Approved Nurse Aide Training Program
  - o State competency test within 24 months of the program's completion through HDmaster

- Texas

  - o State-approved nurse aide training and competency evaluation program
  - o Competency evaluation examination
  - o Entitled to be on the Texas Nurse Aide Registry through waiver or reciprocity

- Utah

- o Approved CNA training program
- o State CNA competency test through HDmaster

- Vermont

  - o Verification of completing a state-approved nursing assistant program
  - o NNAAP examination

- Virginia

  - o Virginia-approved Nurse Aide Training Program
  - o Virginia Nurse Aide written or oral and skills evaluation

- Washington

  - o State-approved program (at least 85 hours of training)
  - o Nursing assistant competency exam

- Washington, DC

  - o Authorized Nurse Aide Training Program (45 hours of classroom teaching, 30 hours of clinics, and 45 hours of nursing home practicums)
  - o Nurse aide examination through Pearson VUE

- West Virginia

  - o Same as Washington, DC

- Wisconsin

  - o Approved Nurse Aide Training Program
  - o Competency test

- Wyoming

  - o State-approved CNA training program
  - o Application and fingerprint cards to the Wyoming State Board of Nursing

o   CNA skills exam via Prometric

National Nurse Aide Assessment Program (NNAAP)

Congress adopted the Nursing Home Reform Act as a component of the Omnibus Budget Reconciliation Act of 1987 (OBRA '87) to augment healthcare in long-term facilities and set nursing training and assessment standards.

Ensuring quality healthcare led to the creation of the National Nurse Assistant Assessment Program (NNAAP®), which examines whether an individual has the minimal competency to become a certified nursing assistant. The program, developed by the National Council of State Boards of Nursing, Inc. (NCSBN), ensures that those certified satisfy the necessary skills, abilities, and knowledge required by federal and state regulations and laws. Pearson VUE, and other authorized agencies like Prometric and HDMaster, conduct the test in different states.

The NNAAP certification allows you to practice in your state. Moving to a different state with another NNAAP requirement will require recertification. However, the same certificate will work if both states accept similar specifications. NNAAP certification sanctions and recommends that you can safely perform as a nurse assistant that clients trust and recognize.

The American Red Cross conducts complete courses for test preparation besides other providers. Renewal of certification every two years depends upon the fulfillment of the following clauses:

- CNAs must work for a state-approved minimum number of hours.
- There is no record of abuse or negligence of duties.
- A requisite number of hours of state-approved mandatory outgoing education.

Structure of CNA Test

The CNA test has two components: a written or oral examination and a skills demonstration test. To obtain CNA certification, passing both parts is a must. It adds your name to the state Nurse Aide Registry.

Written Part of CNA

The written component has 70 multiple-choice questions, a. Of these, ten are non-scoring for gathering statistical information. Otherwise, you can choose an oral examination. It has 60 multiple-choice questions. Ten items are for word recognition and serve as a reading comprehension test. You will listen to recorded questions on a headset. You have to select your answer from a list of given choices. Decide your preferred mode of examination during registration.

The written or oral examination has three segments: Physical Care Skills, Psychosocial Care Skills, and Role of the Nurse Aide. The time allotted for the entire test section is two hours.

Physical Care Skills (with 61% emphasis)

Physical care skills have three sections as follows:

- Daily living activities comprising 14% of the test has nine questions. The topics include hygiene, dressing and grooming, nutrition and hydration, elimination, and rest/sleep/comfort.
- Covering 39% of the test is basic nursing skills with 23 questions. Topics are controlling infection, safety measures during emergencies, therapeutic and technical methods, and data compiling and documentation.
- Restorative skills comprise 8% of a test with five questions—aspects like prevention, self-care, and client independence feature in this test category.

Psychosocial Care Skills (with 13% emphasis)

The two sections of psychosocial care skills are as follows:

- Emotional and mental health needs with six questions cover 11% of the test.
- Spiritual and cultural needs comprise 2% of the test with two questions.

Role of the Nurse Aide (with 26% emphasis)

This category tests whether you have the knowledge and skills as a nurse aide in the following domains:

- Communication with four questions covers 8% of the test.
- The client rights section has four questions with a 7% weightage.
- Legal and ethical conduct has a 3% weight with two questions.
- The member of the health care team covers 8% of the test with five questions.

Clinical Skills Examination

In the skills demonstration section, you must perform five critical skills out of 23 skills. The test setting resembles a potential workplace. A nurse aide evaluator marks your performance. A candidate volunteers as a debilitated older individual. All the necessary tools for carrying out the skills will be present in the test setting.

All skills consist of sequential tasks; a performance measurement depends on the techniques of each task completion. You have 30 minutes to perform this section. Each task has a critical step. You must do it accurately to pass that skill. The skills tested are as follows:

- Hand hygiene
- Applying one knee-high elastic stocking
- Assisting in ambulation using a transfer belt
- Helping with the use of bedpan
- Cleaning of upper or lower dentures
- Counting and recording radial pulse
- Counting and recording respirations
- Donning and removing PPE (gown and gloves)
- Dressing the client with a weak right arm

- Feeding clients who cannot self-feed
- Giving modified bed bath involving the face and one arm, hand, and underarm
- Measuring and recording electronic blood pressure
- Measuring and recording manual blood pressure
- Measuring and recording urinary output
- Measuring and recording the weight of an ambulatory client
- Performing modified passive range of motion (PROM) for one knee and one ankle
- Performing modified passive range of motion (PROM) for one shoulder
- Positioning on side
- Providing catheter care for female
- Providing foot care on one foot
- Providing mouth care
- Providing female perineal care (peri-care)
- Transferring from bed to wheelchair employing a transfer belt.

The official vendors for CNA tests, like Credentia, Pearson VUE, and others, require registration to take the test. Once you select your state, the website directs you to the specific platform for signing with the vendor. After opening an account, the process involves:

- Making new applications.
- Selecting the eligibility route applicable to you.
- Fill in the necessary information.
- Submitting relevant documents the process requires.

An email confirms receipt of the application and its approval. You can now register for the test.

The next step is scheduling written or oral and clinical or lab tests. Choose the test mode, written or oral, and online or on-site in a nearby testing center. If you want to take an online test, you can schedule it until the day before, as long as the exam is still available.

If you choose to take the test at a testing place, sign up at least ten days in advance to ensure you have sufficient time. Pay for the online test with a credit or prepaid credit card—each state issues a candidate's handbook to guide the applicant. Examination fees are approximately $100, with statewide variations.

The number of test questions on theoretical knowledge can vary among testing vendors. The same can be said about the pass scores. Visiting each state's CNA links online is essential to corroborate the facts.

A Prometric conducted test consists of a written test of 90 minutes duration and clinical tests for 31 - 40 minutes, depending on the skills. HDmaster gives 90 minutes to complete the 75-question knowledge test. You receive an alert 15 minutes to time completion. You are not permitted to query about the test content, like, "What is the meaning of this question?"

The Regional Centers of different states also receive applications, supporting documents, and fees, following which they schedule for testing.

Test Day

The event can take up the whole day. Prometric schedules written and skills tests five minutes apart to ensure all candidates are present at the test center. Arrive 15 minutes before the scheduled time. Being late will cancel your test without a refund. Ensure carrying necessary IDs as required by the testing center. They can be as follows:

- Original Social Security card (unlaminated)
- Valid, current government-issued legal photo identification card bearing your signature, like the driver's license
- Requisite supporting documents

You are allowed the following items:

- Watch with a secondhand
- Non-skid footwear
- Dress professionally, preferably in a uniform.
- Two sharpened No. 2 pencils
- Eraser

- A non-electronic language word-for-word translation dictionary must be shown to the knowledge test proctor before starting the knowledge exam

The following are not allowed:

- Cellular phones, beepers, or any other electronic devices
- Personal belongings such as briefcases, large bags, study materials, etc. Eating, drinking, smoking, or taking a break during the exam
- Creating any disturbance or misconduct
- Visitors, guests, pets, or children
- Carrying any test materials out of the examination center

The onboarding procedure by the testing vendors guides you through the correct way to approach the examination.

Test Score

Test results are available online a few hours following the test. You receive an email notification. Certain states physically post the results within five to seven business days.

If you pass both examinations, the state's nursing aide registry will list you a few weeks to months later. If you fail the test, you may make a formal grievance or complaint to the state or retake it.

Some states require a pass score of 70%–75%, while others may require an 80% score. Scoring for the skill test is on each task without omitting the key steps in bold.

PACE Preparation Method

In the nursing profession, fast and efficient decision-making makes significant improvements to patient care. You may know about the skills, but their application to specific situations requires a different approach. For instance, if an older adult complains of constipation, which skill sets must you use or consider? What points should immediately surface in your mind?

Constipation can occur from inadequate food and fluid consumption. You must check for dehydration, feel the skin elasticity, query about the urine output, and monitor fluid intake.

The innovative PACE study method helps you to appraise the profession critically, make capable decisions, and develop an intuition concerning an action. Apply the mnemonic to practice different CNA skills.

- Prepare

    o Review the line of action and understand the sequential nature of the steps of a skill. Concentrate on the critical step and appreciate its importance in linking the other steps.
    o Gather the necessary supplies to perform the skill.
    o Verify patient care plan.

- Assess

    o Assess the patient's condition, ambulatory or immobilized.
    o Ensure patient comfort level.
    o Assess potential procedural risks involved, like damaging a denture while cleaning it.

- Carry out

    o Implement the steps of the procedure.
    o Focus on client safety and comfort.

- Evaluate

    o Monitor the patient's response.
    o Evaluate procedural usefulness.

Summary

- The CNA exam is a certification to become a certified nursing assistant. The CNA exam consists of a written/oral and a clinical skills test.

- A state-approved training program before taking the CNA exam is mandatory.
- A CNA Certification exam is a two-part, multiple-choice test generally taking 2 hours to complete.
- Each state has its passing score on the CNA test varying from 70%–80%.

The next chapter discusses physical care skills, an essential component of knowledge, aptitude, and application of CNA training that you, as a CNA, put into daily practice with mastery.

Chapter Two: Physical Care Skills

The most satisfying part of a nurse's job is to provide physical care to their patients. Nurses tend to the weak and sick individuals. Doing well unto them gives a rare satisfaction and upliftment of spirit that cannot be measured only by financial gains. The faculty of perception that enables you to detect the physical symptoms of a patient, client, or resident to offer them assistance and care is bound to give you 100% job satisfaction.

The PACE method advocates integrating holistic and scientific processes into everyday healthcare to make it top-quality and compassionate. In 1958, Ida Jean Orlando based her nursing care approaches on John Maslow's hierarchy of needs. It emphasizes the basic physical needs that must be satisfied before higher-order goals like self-worth. Nursing care primarily aims to provide physical and emotional care and reliable nursing interventions. Thus, physical care and safety form the fundamental base of Maslow's needs hierarchy (Tony-Butler and Thayer, 2023) and nursing care.

Personal care is unique to a patient and with daily variations. As a CNA, you must be able to decipher the exact care plan you must deliver.

Personal care skills includes the following topics:

- Skincare and preventing pressure sores
- Changing sides and positioning residents

- Denture care
- Controlling contractures
- Assisting patients with impaired vision and hearing
- Feeding residents

Overview of Physical Care Skills

Before going into patient care, knowing the terms that define a nurse assistant's work settings would be helpful. A resident is an individual who receives care in a long-term facility for over six months. They may inhabit the place temporarily or permanently, depending upon their conditions.

A long-term care facility gives medical, personal, and social assistance to residents over a prolonged period. It is of two types: nursing homes and assisted-living facilities. The latter offers its residents assistance with activities of daily living (ADLs) like bathing, feeding, or moving around the facility. Some are independent and only require help with some aspects of living, like reminders to take medications.

Those living in nursing homes depend more on care services and need supervision. Nursing home residents are mostly older people with one or more chronic conditions; some can be younger people suffering from medical conditions or mental health illnesses. A disease is considered chronic when it persists for a prolonged period or is incurable but can be controlled (American Red Cross Nurse Assistant Training, 2012).

Most residents of nursing homes require assistance with ADLs. Chronic conditions, such as arthritis, heart or lung diseases, can further incapacitate the patients. They may need help getting in and out of bed, eating, taking medicines, or using the toilet.

Physical ailments have mental repercussions. They can make people feel lonely and hopeless. A nurse assistant can reassure them with their supportive actions. Patients can find solace in their compassionate words.

Patients can also choose to receive home care. People who opt for this service are called clients. Home healthcare agencies provide care services for sub-acute or chronic cases, shifting clients to hospitals only in emergencies, acute illnesses, or accidents. Clients can also be sub-par with their ADLs but are not prepared to shift to a long-term care facility.

Nurse assistants working in home settings are called home health aides. They work under a licensed nurse and report to them. However, they visit the client's home independently and assist in preparing meals, personal care, and light household tasks. Home health aides must be able to work independently and comfortably; help is not readily available. The core functioning qualities are flexibility and adjustability. Also, a home may not have gadgets readily available in a care facility.

Communication is the most significant quality for a nurse assistant in any setting. It is one of the six care principles.

Six Principles of Care

The six care principles suggested by the Red Cross are dignity, safety, infection control, communication, independence, and privacy.

Dignity: Face the patient while communicating with them whenever applicable. Speak clearly and use the patient's name while addressing them.

Safety: Hippocrates, the father of medicine, is often quoted as saying, "First, do no harm." And it is no surprise that he mentioned it in his work, *Of the Epidemics*. Safety ensures the containment of infections, prevention of accidents and falls, and protects clients and staff. Safety includes installing call lights, side rails, non-slippery mats, using apt body maneuvers, and providing warmth. Before addressing an individual, check the ID band and greet them using this name.

Infection control: Wearing gloves and personal protective equipment (PPE), applying the correct procedure of donning and doffing PPE, disposing of used materials and gear, changing soiled linens and making beds, and using barrier nursing are all aspects of infection control.

Nursing assistants need to **communicate** effectively with varying personalities throughout the day. They can be patients, family members, supervisors, or other staff members. Introducing yourself using your proper name and stating your designations with a smile establishes a quick affinity with others. It encourages trust and ensures comfortable interactions.

As a CNA, you must prioritize and value the patient's **independence** in making decisions and allowing you to carry out specific tasks. Seek permission before any procedure using non-medical words. Motivate decision-making capacities and self-care habits in patients whenever feasible.

Various ways can ensure patient **privacy**. Knock on the door before entering and then close the door behind you. Pull the curtain around the bed to segregate the patient from others before you do a procedure on them. Draping to cover body parts not under intervention gives patients much-needed privacy and protection.

Activities of Daily Living

As CNAs, you will be crucial in providing patients under your care with adequate and correct nutrition and hydration. Many older adults have type 2 diabetes, liver diseases, or heart conditions preventing them from having specific food items. Patients with kidney disorders may need fluid restrictions. A CNA must follow medical instructions, assist patients with personal care, help select appropriate clothing, use the bathroom, and move around the facility.

Basic Nursing Skills

Basic nursing skills are embedded in the nursing profession. Just as a driver knows how to turn a car right, you must know how to do certain things related to patient care. Some examples are as follows:

- Knowing when to weigh the patient (same time every day)
- The correct method of recording oral temperature (waiting for 15 minutes if the patient has had a cold drink to allow the oral cavity to return to average temperature)

- Correct procedure of discarding gowns and gloves after seeing an infected patient (leave the items in the current patient's room before caring for another patient to prevent the spread of infection to other staff and patients)

Accurately recording weight, vital signs, and blood pressure; confidence with ADLs; and sound knowledge of infection control procedures are some primary nursing duties typical to all healthcare settings.

Restorative Skills

Restorative skills are nursing activities that enable the resident to operate as independently as possible. For instance, a resident may want to spend the day in a wheelchair despite the assistance of physical therapists. It delays the recovery process.

A CNA's commitment to preserving the resident's regained function encourages and supports the resident, urging them to walk. Providing emotional and psychological support in addition to physical treatment makes it even more therapeutic.

Daily preventative care may help avoid difficulties caused by inactivity, inadequate nutrition, and skin deterioration from toileting issues. In that aspect, restorative skills go one step beyond rehabilitation to fortify it.

Some examples of restorative skills include knowing the "passive" range of muscle movements. It means you must support the patient's arm while carefully circulating it around its range of motions.

Activities of Daily Living

Activities of daily living (ADLs) help us to maintain self-care, keeping us healthy and fit. It can be **basic** but essential tasks like bathing, grooming, feeding, or using the toilet. **Instrumental** ADLs are tasks that an individual must be able to perform to live independently. They are shopping, cooking, cleaning, having timely medicines, and managing finances.

Different types of ADLs are as follows:

- Grooming
- Hygiene

  o Mobility and toileting
  o Immobility

- AM care
- PM care
- Basic vs. Instrumental
- Ambulation
- Range of motion
- Feeding

  o Nutrition

Grooming

Grooming means caring for personal hygiene to keep the body clean and tidy. It involves shaving, combing, teeth and nail care, etc.

Hair Care

- Hair care involves brushing, combing, and hair styling
- Communicate with patients regarding their preferences.
- Use gentle movements and close observation of facial features for expressions of pain or discomfort. Report the following:

  o Sores on the person's scalp
  o Atypical flaking or dandruff
  o Undue hair loss
  o Tangles that cannot be drawn out

- Shampooing
- Shaving

o Carefully shave patients to prevent scratches and infections
o Use electric razors to reduce the chances of accidents
o Avoid manual razors for safety issues

Dressing and Undressing

- It gives identity and purpose.
- Minimal change of clothes during the daytime and before bed. Additionally, clothing needs changing if it is soiled or wet.
- Choose more manageable clothing for the person to wear and take off.
- Encourage patients not acutely ill to dress and undress themselves using assisted devices if necessary.
- Consider the following while selecting clothing:

  o Individual choices
  o Physical capabilities
  o Day's activities
  o The climate and the season

Manicure and Pedicure

- Nail care to contain infections from scratching
- Sterile materials and hand hygiene
- Special care for nail care for diabetic patients

Oral Care

- Distinct techniques for conscious and unconscious patients
- Appropriate oral care kit
- Periodic oral care to prevent infections
- Indications of infection

Bathing

- Ensure bathing safety. Use assistive devices to avert accidents.

- Check skin breaks and scratches to avoid infections.
- Privacy during bathing.
- Observe and report skin ailments or bed sores.

Feeding

Clients may need assistance opening food packages, settling down with their meals, or eating food. Some essential nursing activities are as follows:

- Wash hands before beginning the procedure.
- Sit at the client's eye level and use napkins to protect clothing.
- Deliver bite-sized morsels with a spoon.
- Allow the client to chew and swallow their mouthful before offering the next.
- Offer fluid after each three or four bites.
- Use this time to interact with the client, making mealtimes a positive experience.
- Encourage meal completion but do not enforce it when they refuse or are full.
- Note and report any problems with eating or persistent refusals to the nurse in charge.

Ambulation

The need for assistance with movement or ambulation is unique for each client. Clients can be safely transferred between places using the commonly applied assisted device, a gait-transfer belt.

- Tie the belt firmly around the client's waist. Position yourself in front of the client. Keep your legs slightly apart.
- Hold the gait belt with both hands and help the client to stand with their feet between yours.
- Once the client is ready, transfer one hand to the belt's side and the other to the back. Walk with the client, supporting them with the belt at the side or back.

- Do not catch or prevent the client from falling if they tumble. Instead, bend your knees and softly drop the client to the floor, supporting the head and letting them rest on your leg. Call for assistance and stay with the client to avoid further injuries.

Range of Movement (ROM)

Perform the range of movement exercises on clients in the following manner:

- Position the client comfortably supine (flat) on his back.
- Initiate the procedure by performing smooth circular (rotation) shoulder motions, first one, then another, and then moving them toward (adducting) and away (abducting) from the client's body.
- Bend (flex) and straighten (extend) the lower arms with your hands supporting the client's elbows and wrists.
- Make circular motions to the wrists and extend each hand, finger, and thumb.
- Supporting the foot and ankle, flex each leg from the knee.
- Adduct, abduct, and rotate each leg at the hip joint.
- Support each foot's instep, rotate, flex, and extend it at the ankle. Then, flex and extend the toes.
- Avoid using force on a limb (extremity) that feels tense or stiffened.
- Report any atypical observations to the RN promptly.

Hygiene

Hygiene is maintaining physical cleanliness and minimizing the spread of disease by regular self-care routines. The main purpose is preventing infectious diseases from occurring.

Mobility and Toileting

- Aid patients with toileting. Maintain self-respect.
- Observe toileting routines, significantly for senior patients.

- Report defecation promptly.

Clients with restricted mobility may use a bedside commode or bedpan rather than going to the bathroom. Observe the following while assisting a client with toileting:

- The commode must be locked, and the client must be as close to it as possible.
- Check toilet paper and other items in hand.
- Encourage privacy but not at the cost of safety.
- Place a protective pad under the client if they ask for a bedpan. For a client in a position to shift, roll them to one side to place the pan under the buttocks. Raise the head end of the bed to make the client sit up and lower it once finished. Remove the pan, clean, and wipe dry the perineal region.
- Throughout the procedure, maintain client dignity, safety, and maximum possible privacy.

Immobility

Clients can be mobile and able to self-care to an extent. Some can be immobile and need assistance with personal hygiene. They regularly receive cleansing bed baths. Although facilities can use branded waterless shampoo and bathing wipes, regular soap and water for cleansing is also feasible. The following are the steps of a partial bed bath:

- The water must be comfortable.
- Uncover only the body part you are cleaning, and wipe the area promptly with a clean towel.
- Use a wet washcloth for the face. Wipe the eyes from the inner to outer canthus (corner of the eyes at the junction of upper and lower lids) with its clean part.
- Apply some soap to the washcloth to wipe the rest of the body.
- Turn the client on their side and wipe the back and the back of the extremities.
- Apply warm lotion on the skin and change the client into fresh clothes and gowns.
- Observe any sign of skin rashes or cracks and report to the nurse.

AM Care

AM care involves the following activities:

- Toileting, changing soiled (incontinence) undergarments, and giving perineal (space between the anus and scrotum in males and the anus and the vulva in females) care
- Oral (mouth) and denture care, depending on residents' preferences
- Depending on residents' schedule, partial bath, full bath, or shower
- Dressing or changing the hospital gown
- Grooming, such as hair care, shaving, and applying makeup, accessories, or jewelry according to residents' preferences
- Helping with eating breakfast
- Giving timely hand hygiene to the resident
- Helping with activities, physical therapy (PT), and occupational therapy (OT)
- Bed-making and organizing the resident's room

PM Care

PM care involves the following tasks:

- Toileting
- Helping with lunch and dinner
- Partial bath, full bath, or shower, depending on the residents' schedule
- Oral and denture care before bed
- Oral care after meals if a resident prefers
- Wash the face and remove any makeup
- Change into a gown or pajamas
- Offering hand hygiene as needed
- Organizing the resident's room

Basic Nursing Skills

Since caring for patients is at the core of nursing, nurse assistants must have a solid foundation of nursing abilities and knowledge to do their jobs efficiently. As a CNA, you must understand nursing principles, including patient assessment, vital sign measurement, care planning, and diagnostic and treatment assistance. A thorough comprehension of medical language and legal and ethical principles is critical to your role.

The skills include the following:

- Preventing infection from flaring
- Technical approaches
- Common conditions of the residents
- Vital signs
- Safety
- Basic medical and health knowledge

    o Anatomy
    o Biological systems

- Response to emergencies

    o Breathing emergencies
    o Burns
    o Chest pain
    o Hemorrhage
    o Loss of consciousness
    o Seizures

- Stroke
- Trauma
- Natural catastrophes

    o Tornado
    o Thunderstorm
    o Power outage

Infection

Whether you serve a patient in a hospital, nursing home, long-term facility, or at home, as a certified nursing assistant, you will always be obligated to ensure your patients' health and well-being. Of primary concern is preventing the spread of infection. Infection is caused by microscopic organisms (microbes) like bacteria, viruses, yeast, or parasites. They enter the body through broken skin, airways, mouth, ears, urinary and genital tracts. Harmful microbes that cause infection are pathogens.

Common symptoms of infection are as follows:

- Fever
- Red or pus-filled eyes
- Pus-filled nasal discharge
- Cough
- Headache
- Sore throat
- Loss of appetite
- Nausea
- Stomach ache
- Diarrhea
- Vomiting
- Cloudy or malodorous urine
- Joint pain
- Muscle ache
- Skin rash
- Sores
- Redness and swelling around a wound
- Wound with pus

Senior adults with co-existing diseases like diabetes or stroke may not manifest overt symptoms of infection. Its subtle symptoms can be as follows:

- Newly developed or worsening confusion
- Appetite or eating pattern changes
- Newly developed or worsening bladder and bowel incontinence
- Lack of coherence
- Fatigue
- Flu-like symptoms

Infections that spread from one to another are communicable diseases. Some examples are common cold, whooping cough, strep throat, gastroenteritis, pink eye, gonorrhea, hepatitis B, HIV, and warts.

- Prevent communicable diseases through good hygiene like handwashing, sanitizers, and PPEs.
- Ensure items once used for a patient are correctly discarded.
- Each person must have their items.
- Handle used linens carefully. Linens must not touch your uniform. Use PPE when handling used or soiled linen.
- Dispose of linen according to the policies of the facility.
- Wash used linen adequately with hot water and detergent, and store them in a clean, dry place.
- Vaccines can prevent many communicable diseases like influenza, Covid-19, and hepatitis A and B.
- Cover bedpans and urinals.
- Prepare food hygienically.
- Serve meals directly.
- Store foods properly.
- If you are sick, stay at home.

Common Resident Conditions

- Arthritis
- Diarrhea
- Fever
- Urinary tract infections
- Respiratory tract infections like pneumonia and influenza
- Gastroenteritis
- Skin infection
- Sepsis

- Dementia

Vital Signs

A CNA's routine task includes taking and recording a patient's vital signs. They provide valuable information about the functioning of an individual's body systems. Procedural inaccuracy can vastly alter results, impairing proper diagnosis. The vital signs are as follows:

- Body temperature
- Respiration
- Pulse
- Blood pressure

Safety

- Medical and Surgical Asepsis:

    o Medical asepsis eliminates disease-producing microorganisms.
    o Proper hand hygiene using soap and water or alcohol-based hand rubs provides medical asepsis.
    o Surgical asepsis keeps equipment sterile during interventions.
    o Maintain sterility while donning PPE comprising gloves, masks, goggles, gowns, head and shoe coverings.

- Sharps Care and Discarding

    o Sharps are sharp-edged and pointed medical appliances like needles and syringes.
    o Wear gloves. Avoid recapping or bending needles.
    o Ensure proper sharps disposal in FDA-cleared containers.
    o For accidental pricks, wash the area, use antiseptic, and attend medical treatment.

- Equipment Handling

    o Ensure a safe, sanitized hospital environment.
    o Promptly remove and clean of small blood or fluid spillage with appropriate cleaning fabrics.

- o Ensure proper storing of sterilized equipment and discarding of used or waste items.
- o Sterilize endoscopes after each use.

- **Resident Safety**:

  - o Ensure a safe patient environment by stemming falls, confirming medication administration, inspecting electrical openings, and knowing fire safety protocols.
  - o Monitor patients for shifts in movement, bowel habits, looks, activity status, vital signs, appetite, and sleeping patterns.
  - o Report any problems to the supervisor promptly.

Basic Medical and Health Knowledge

Knowing human anatomy and physiology is foundational to the nursing profession. Human anatomy consists of different systems that we will briefly delineate here.

Skeletal System

The skeletal or musculoskeletal system provides a supportive framework for the human body. An adult skeleton comprises 206 bones. The functions of the skeletal system are as follows:

- Supporting posture, gait, and balance
- Protection of internal organs

  - o Skull: brain
  - o Vertebra: spinal cord
  - o Sternum (breastbone) and 12 Ribs: Lungs and the heart
  - o Pelvis: lower parts of urinary and digestive systems and genital organs

- Production of red and white blood cells in the red marrow
- Storing minerals like calcium, phosphorus, etc.

Conditions that affect this system are:

- Arthritis is the decaying of bone structures, resulting in pain, stiffness, and joint immobility. Factors leading to arthritis are age, trauma, and medical conditions like Lyme disease or immunological disorders.
- Fracture is breaking bones due to injury, stress, diseases like osteoporosis and rickets, tumors, and mechanical stress.
- Osteoporosis is the loss of bones, making them fragile and brittle due to lack of calcium.
- Sprains and tears due to age, diseases, and injuries.

Some important bones are:

- Skull
- Collar bones: the clavicle (2)
- Shoulder blades: the scapula (2)
- Ribs (12)
- Breastbone: the sternum (1)
- Spinal column: the vertebral Column (1)
- Tailbone: the coccyx (1)
- Forearm: the humerus (2)
- Lower arm: radius and ulna (1 each on each side)
- Pelvis
- Upper leg: the femur (2)
- Lower leg: tibia and fibula (1 each on each side)
- Smallest bones: the ossicles (inner ear)
- The largest bone: the femur.

Long bones, such as the limbs, have marrow-filled center cavities. Young bones have red marrows, and aging marrow is primarily fat cells called yellow marrow.

Organ Systems

The human body depends on the efficient functioning of the various organ systems for its survival, like food digestion and elimination of wastes, distribution of nutrients, and conduction of senses and movement. These systems are:

- Nervous System
- Cardiovascular System
- Respiratory System
- Digestive System
- Urinary System
- Reproductive System
- Skin

Nervous System

We engage with the internal and external world through the mechanics of the nervous system. It consists of the following:

- Central Nervous System (CNS)

  o Cognition, emotions, memory, and sensory receptor data processing occur in the **brain**, the "clearing house" for all information. It coordinates all bodily functions, which cannot survive otherwise without artificial help. It is bathed in cerebrospinal fluid (CSF).
  o **The spinal cord** comprises a bundle of nerve fibers that carry information to and from the brain to the rest of the body.

- Peripheral Nervous System

  o **Nerves** from the brain (12) and spinal cord (31) transmit sensory receptor data to the CNS for processing. The CNS commands the body via peripheral nerves. Nerve cells are called neurons—their number declines after age 25.

Cardiovascular System

The cardiovascular system comprises the following:

Heart: The right side receives deoxygenated blood from the body through the veins. It pumps this blood to the lungs to enrich it with oxygen. Oxygenated blood comes to the left side and is distributed to the body via the arteries.

Lungs: detoxify blood containing CO2 and replace it with oxygen. We inhale (breathe in) to take oxygen and exhale (breathe out) to release CO2. Air exchange occurs in the smallest sac-like lung structures, called alveoli. Air passes up and down through the airways consisting of the bronchioles, bronchi (si. bronchus), the trachea (windpipe), and the nasal passages.

Blood vessels: Arteries break into a fine meshwork of capillaries to bathe the tissues and supply them with nutrients and oxygen. The veins collect the waste from the capillary network.

Blood

The functions of the cardiovascular system are as follows:

- Blood circulation.
- Maintain temperature and blood pressure.
- Carry oxygen from the lungs to the body.
- Carry CO2 from the body to the lungs to be eliminated.
- Transport nutrients for processing and distribution.

Respiratory problems like chronic bronchitis and pneumonia are commonly found in senior people. Common heart conditions include hypertension, rhythm disturbances, thickened arterial walls, and cardiac ailments. Orthostatic hypotension or fall in blood pressure on postural changes (standing up from a seated or supine position) occurs due to loss of blood vessel elasticity.

Digestive System

The digestive system extends from the mouth to the anus. Its structures are as follows:

- Pharynx: is common to food and oxygen. Air enters the trachea and the lungs from here, while food passes into the esophagus.
- Esophagus
- Stomach
- Small intestine
- Large intestine

- Rectum
- Liver
- Gallbladder

The liver, a right-sided structure, is located beneath the rib cage. It and the gall bladder are part of the digestive system and aid digestion and assimilation of nutrients. Alcohol and drug abuse can damage the liver.

The gallbladder is a sac-like structure below the liver. It secretes and stores bile. Stones in the gallbladder and inflammation can necessitate its removal. Affected individuals must be careful with their diet and take supplements.

The functions of the liver are as follows:

- Produce cholesterol.
- Filter toxins from the blood.
- Secrete bile that helps in digestion.
- Control blood sugar.
- Produce vital immunological elements.

Urinary System

The urinary system eliminates waste products in the form of urine. Adults produce approximately a quart and a half of urine daily. The quantity of food and fluid consumed daily and the amount lost through sweating and breathing determines urine volume. Kidneys, like the liver, eliminate medicine byproducts. Their damage can cause drug toxicity.

The urinary system comprises the following structures:

- Kidney (2) filters the blood of toxins and chemicals and forms urine. It maintains fluid and electrolyte balance. Kidneys release a small quantity of urine that passes through the ureters to the urinary bladder.
- Ureters (2)
- Urinary Bladder (1) collects urine until a pressure sensation urges us to urinate.

Urea, a waste like CO_2, is a byproduct of protein, poultry, and some vegetables like spinach digestion. Blood carries urea to the kidneys into urine. Excess urea can accumulate in tissue, causing an inflammatory condition called gout.

As a nursing assistant, helping patients empty their bladders is crucial. Patients frequently phone or text you when they need to use the bathroom while you're working. Patients have more trouble controlling bladder urges than usual, so waiting more than a few minutes may be challenging.

When patients cannot promptly empty their bladder in the toilet or with a bedpan, it can be a humiliating accident for them. Also, accumulated urine can cause urinary tract infection (UTI). Urine receding into the kidneys can cause kidney infection. It raises patient suffering and needs prescription drugs. The risk of future incontinence may increase.

Skin

Skin, the body's largest organ, is stretched over a large surface area. It serves the following functions:

- Keeping organs in position.
- Protecting delicate organs.
- Regulating body moisture and temperature.
- Protecting the body from infection.

Older adults lose skin elasticity and efficiency of temperature regulation. Conversely, some medications can decrease sweat production (atropine) and raise body temperature. As CNAs, you must watch your patients' skin for breakages, wounds, elasticity, and moisture. Maintaining skin hydration and health is vital to nursing care.

Emergencies

Emergency measures are immediate actions that save the patient's life and fatal consequences (Emergency Response for CNA and HHA, 2022).

- Burns

  - o Smother the flames with a large blanket or ask the patient to roll on the ground.
  - o Provide first aid with cool, running water for 20 minutes.
  - o Avoid repeating as the effect persists for three hours.
  - o Keep the patient warm.
  - o Avoid toothpaste, butter, oil, eggs, turmeric, or ice.

- Hemorrhage

  - o Apply direct pressure to the bleeding site.
  - o Arterial bleed pumps out blood. If unstopped, hemorrhage leads to rapid blood loss and death. Apply a tourniquet above an arm or leg bleed.

- Unconsciousness

  - o Secure airways, check breathing, pulse, and blood pressure.
  - o Wait for the EMS to arrive.
  - o Spontaneous recovery can happen. Still, underlying heart or nervous system problems may be present.

- Seizures

  - o Generalized convulsions affect the whole body. Other seizures can seem like lapses in conversation, confusion, and aimless movements like facial twitches, vacant looks, and wringing of hands.
  - o Lay the patient on the floor. Loosen the garments. Move things that can hurt the patient. Avoid restraining the patient.
  - o Convulsions last for one or two minutes, then confusion and gradual awareness.
  - o Patients with recurrent convulsions understand when to call EMS.
  - o Need for EMS

    - First-time seizure activity

- Unstoppable convulsions
- Impaired respiration
- Not regaining consciousness

- Stroke

    o Patients with stroke can have cerebrovascular or cardiovascular accidents. They are unaware of problems and unable to judge an action course.
    o Call 911 in doubtful situations. Time is crucial for survival.
    o Urgent use of thrombolytics can prevent permanent disability due to damage by blood clots.
    o Symptoms include

    - Unilateral numbness or weakness of the face, arm, or leg
    - Confusion, slurred speech, problems with speech comprehension
    - Visual disturbances
    - Dizziness, coordination loss
    - Severe, atypical headache

- Trauma

    o Avoid moving the individual unless critical. Forcing an individual with spinal injuries can cause paralysis.
    o Stop any bleeding.

- Chest pain
- In middle-aged males, chest pain can have the following features:

    o Pain (heaviness, burning, choking, or squeezing) behind the sternum. Patients show the area by placing a fist over the sternum.
    o Sweating, cold, and clammy skin
    o Nausea or vomiting
    o Shortness of breath
    o Lightheadedness
    o Anxiety with raised heart rate
    o Pain below the ribs, back, neck, jaw, or shoulders

o   History of recent exercise, eating, cold exposure, or emotional stress. Chest pain in females, older people, and people with diabetes lack these features.

o   A CNA's job is to ensure the following:

- Note the characteristics and location of chest pain. Take patient history and drug history if possible.
- Seek help and assemble devices (AED, defibrillator, crash cart, and oxygen).
- Monitor vital signs
- Give oxygen.

- Sudden breathing difficulties can be fast or shallow breathing, sudden cough, or coughing blood. The following steps can help:

o   Perform the Heimlich maneuver if the patient has choked on food.

o   When a patient is on oxygen, check its flow. Bluishness of lips and mucosa and nail bed (cyanosis) indicates a lack of oxygen.

Natural Disasters

Preparations for a disaster need proactive planning and organization in any healthcare setting. Emergency supplies include flashlights, extra batteries, drinking water, packaged food items, blankets, and first-aid kits. Hospitals have backup power supplies like generators. All electronic equipment, like ventilators, cardiac monitors, IV pumps, bed cords, etc., must be connected to these power supplies. For a home setting, a neighborhood shelter or family member's residence can provide a short-term stay during a power outage.

Tornado

- Ensure everyone is indoors, away from doors and windows.
- When a tornado is spotted, everyone should move down to the lowest floor or the center of the facility under a strong structure until the tornado has receded.

- Facilities in a tornado-prone area must provide tornado guidance and drills.

Thunderstorms

- Everyone must stay inside and away from doors and windows because thunderstorms are associated with lightning that can strike ten miles from a storm.
- Avoid using electrical devices like landline telephones or computers plugged into a power outlet.
- Patients must be out of bathtubs, pools, and showers as lightning can pass through water bodies.

Power Outage

- Check emergency provisions and clean drinking water.
- Storage quality of food refrigerators deteriorates after four to six hours of power outage. Avoid opening the doors of these appliances unnecessarily.
- Food in freezers stays cold for a day or two. Keep all perishable items in the freezer. Discard all items if the temperature climbs over 40°F.
- Patients need warm blankets and clothing layers for winter power outages. Hot summers increase the demand for water and fluids for hydration. Patients need loose-fitting cotton clothes. For extreme heat, use cool clothes for armpits and forehead to bring down temperature.

Restorative Skills

Beyond all typical CNA activities, CNA's multifaceted role entails some competence in restorative abilities. Knowledge of basic medical care and rehabilitation techniques and the time CNAs spend with patients makes them invaluable as primary healthcare providers.

Restorative skills assist clients with preventive care. CNAs motivate their clients to health self-advocacy by offering direct restorative care, ranging from emotional and physical assistance. It helps in achieving their healing goals.

The fundamental aspects of restorative care are as follows:

- Observation
- Inspirational and physical support
- Patience, respect, and optimism
- Basic care like toileting, hygiene, etc.
- Saving resources and complications

How is restorative therapy preventative? Consider the following aspects of the therapy:

- Patient observation for status alteration and immediate reporting to initiate likely interventions can ward off infections or immobility.
- Restoration and maintenance of the physical skills of a patient can enable the highest level of functioning.
- Positive emotional motivation and assistance to inspire patients to assume care for their health as much as possible.
- Feeding, assistance with toileting, and turning immobile patients can prevent many costly complications and are essentially remedial.

The Omnibus Budget and Reconciliation Act (OBRA) of 1987 mandates the following:

- All long-term facilities must use every resource to maintain their residents' best possible physical, psychological, and mental functioning.
- All residents are entitled to make as many decisions as possible concerning lifestyle routines, care, and health.
- Care guidelines must include self-care and independence, which help attain the letter of the law and the spirit of the law in a safe, comforting, and supportive environment.

Mobility & Immobility

Mobility is the ability to move independently, walk, and exercise to maintain muscle mass, balance, and healthy mind and body functions. Lack of mobility or immobility affects various body functions as follows:

- Circulatory system: increased possibility of blood clots (thrombi) and edema of the lower extremities, loading the heart.

- Increased possibility of pneumonia, aspiration, and lung collapse can happen.
- Lack of appetite (anorexia) and constipation.
- Loss of calcium in the bones (osteopenia), muscle wasting (atrophy), and contractures (limb deformities due to immobility) can occur. Bones become brittle (osteoporosis) and liable to fractures.
- Skin ulcers at pressure points.
- Psychological impacts include depression, hopelessness, feelings of isolation, and fears of losing autonomy.
- Social effects include social isolation and poor self-esteem.

Transferring is shifting an immobile patient from one position to another using proper body mechanics and devices like a gait belt. To maintain mobility, CNAs can use the following methods:

- Assisting residents with ROM (free movements of all limbs and joints)
- Passive range of motion exercises (PROM) for immobile individuals
- Movements include
- Abduction (moving limbs away from the body)
- Adduction (moving limbs toward the body)
- Flexion (folding the limbs at their joints)
- Extension (extending the limbs at the joints)
- Reporting and documenting PROM procedures and responses to bolster rehabilitative efforts.
- Following methods to transfer, lift, or move immobile residents:

  o Proper body mechanics
  o Explanation of the procedure
  o Involving the resident in the process
  o Both hands for lifting patients without twisting at the waist
  o The entire body transfer includes moving the top, torso, and legs
  o Logrolling is moving the whole body from side to side
  o Additional help
  o Mechanical lift, lift sheet, etc, for safety

- Positioning devices like hand rolls, wedges, splints, shoes, or boots for dorsiflexion (toes pointed toward the knee) and to prevent contractures, pressure ulcers, and discomfort in immobile patients
- Examples of body positioning include

  o Prone
  o Supine
  o Sim's position
  o Fowler's position

Health maintenance and restoration imply measuring vital signs, height, and weight.

- Factors affecting vital signs are

  o Age
  o Gender
  o Time of the day
  o Illness
  o Emotions
  o Activity
  o Exercise
  o Food intake
  o Medications
  o Change in one parameter (increased heart and respiration rates with >101°F fever)
  o The guidelines for measuring vital signs are

    - Explanation of the procedure
    - Arrange the things required for measurement to make the process efficient and energy-conserving
    - Delay recording oral temperature for 15 minutes after drinking hot fluids

- For weighing a resident, consider

  o Clothing

o   Shoes
o   Time of the day
o   Report notable changes that may mean

- Nutritional deficiency
- Fluid retention
- Significant illness

- Height measurement can indicate changes in posture due to musculo-skeletal problems. Measure height

o   On admission
o   Annually or per facility requirements

Practice Questions

1.   What is the maximum time allotted for a tub bath?

   A. 45 minutes
   B. 30 minutes
   C. 20 minutes
   D. 10 minutes

2.   How would you clean the client's dentures?

   A. Every day
   B. As often as natural teeth
   C. Once a week
   D. Thrice a day

3.   For washing a client's chest during a bed bath, how must CNAs do it?

   A. Cover the chest with a washcloth.
   B. Bare the chest and wash it.
   C. Give a quick wet rub from the neck to the abdomen.
   D. Place a towel over the chest and wash it while lifting the towel slightly.

4.   How long do you soak the foot in warm water for a foot bath?

   A. 10–15 mts
   B. 5–10 mts
   C. 25–30 mts
   D. 1–2 mts

5.   What is the last step of perineal care for uncircumcised males?

   A. Apply moisturizer to the foreskin.
   B. Wash the perineum in a circular motion.
   C. Return the foreskin to its normal state.
   D. Apply dressing to the penis.

6.   What is the first step to oral care?

      A. Maintain privacy.
      B. Adjust the overbed table.
      C. Brushing the teeth.
      D. Flossing the teeth.

7.   What is the best way to remove dentures for cleaning?

      A. Use four fingers and a gloved hand to remove the dentures.
      B. Ask the client to spit the denture into a denture cup.
      C. Remove using a piece of gauze to prevent the denture from slipping.
      D. Ask the client to spit it into your hand.

8.   What is the time for oral hygiene?

      A. Before bathing.
      B. Before breakfast.
      C. After bath.
      D. It depends on the client's care plan.

9.   How to clean the penis during perineal care?

      A. From the urethra
      B. By rubbing vigorously
      C. Using alcohol rub
      D. For one minute

10.   Who determines a hygienic bath for an upset Alzeihmer's patient?

      A. The CNA
      B. The charge nurse
      C. The doctor
      D. The physical therapist

Answers

1. C. Any longer time can chill the client.

2. B. Cleaning dentures should have the same routine as cleaning natural teeth.

3. D. Put a towel over the client's chest, then wash the area while raising the cloth slightly.

4. B. Soaking feet for 5–10 minutes is optimum.

5. C. The final step is returning the foreskin to its normal position.

6. A. Maintaining privacy while giving ADLs is of prime concern.

7. C. Use a piece of gauze to prevent the dentures from slipping.

8. D. Oral care should follow the patient's routine and care plan.

9. A. Cleaning should begin from the urethra to prevent the spread of infections.

10. B. The charge nurse makes all assessments regarding the patient's care and decides accordingly.

PACE Method

The PACE method helps you in your performance strategically. We will discuss providing nail care to patients to explore how this method can help us with every CNA skill we come across. Systemically practicing the techniques will make them your second habit.

- Prepare everything you need for the procedure, like a basin, nail clippers, a jug of warm water, and a towel.

- Assess the nails for infections, fungal or bacterial, bruises, cyanosis, and clubbing. These may indicate underlying conditions like diabetes, circulatory problems, respiratory diseases, or tumors. Check for special orders before carrying out the procedure.
- Carry out the procedure carefully, soaking the nails in lukewarm water for 10–20 minutes, drying them, and clipping them with nail clippers.
- Evaluate your performance and notice if there are any bruises, sharp edges, or skin conditions. Document your findings and report any new or significant problems to the change nurse.

Summary

- Physical care skills include activities of daily living, basic nursing skills, and restorative care skills.
- The six principles of care are maintaining the patient's dignity, infection control, safety, effective communication and listening, independence, and privacy.
- ADLs concern basic hygiene, grooming, feeding, ambulating, and performing a range of motion activities.
- Basic nursing skills are techniques used to prevent infection, measure vital signs, assess common health problems, and ensure safety.
- Basic nursing skills require knowledge of human anatomy and physiology, emergency care, and managing patient care during natural disasters.
- Restorative skills maintain the patient's physical and emotional health, over and above rehabilitative care.
- The PACE method helps prepare, assess, execute, and evaluate care performances.

The next chapter discusses psychosocial care skills that have an overarching effect on the patient's well-being and functionality.

Chapter Three: Psychosocial Care Skills

Mental health is not merely the absence of mental disorders; it is a continuum state of ability to cope with life's stresses, attain the optimum level of our potentialities per circumstances, and contribute to the community. Mental health is integral to a patient's well-being and essential to CNAs' work. Its relevance is in the following areas:

- Understanding patients' emotional challenges
- Offering inspiration and encouragement to enliven the therapeutic process
- Networking with others

The psychosocial section of a CNA test asks questions on the emotional, cultural, and spiritual aspects of the nursing profession. This chapter covers these sections, highlighting the psychosocial care skills component a CNA must have the proficiency to be a skilled worker.

The bearing of psychosocial care services to improve understanding of mental health needs and strengthen health empowerment cannot be undermined. Treatments become more acceptable when patients receive the emotional and mental support of their caregivers, notably the nurses. CNAs, like all other healthcare professionals, must recognize discrimination related to mental illness and attempt to resolve this social injustice as much as possible.

Overview of Psychosocial Care Skills

Basic caregiving is incomplete without ensuring a patient's emotional and mental safety and well-being. Stress and worry accompany physical discomfort and incapacitation. Many fear the changes one must face with aging and infirmity.

As long-time accompaniments and knowledgeable individuals in healthcare segments, CNAs are expected by patients and their families to alleviate fear and tension. They may not write prescriptions, but they are essential to healing because of the care they provide. Care can imbue patients with hope, worth, love, and security. Therefore, even partial care has physical, emotional, and social components.

Emotional Needs

CNAs are more than assistants and listeners; they are champions and grief managers. They are responsible for providing a soothing atmosphere at the hospital and assisting patients with their emotional struggles.

Emotional and mental health, from a social perspective, is the ability to cope with life changes and make adjustments to grief, loss, and loneliness. Erik Erikson's psychosocial developmental stages consider older adulthood from 65 years onward to be when an individual should be able to accept their lives and find fulfillment in their accomplishments and relationships (Mcleod, 2023). Else, it can lead to despair, remorse, and fear of losing control over life. Also, changes can add to mental stress. Feelings of abandonment, loss of freedom, and resentment can cause irritability, depression, or suicidal ideation. Neurological, cardiovascular, or musculoskeletal disorders can add to psychosocial problems.

CNAs can help patients emotionally in the following manner:

- Practicing compassion and consideration for each individual in all forms of communication, verbal and nonverbal
- Listening with patience and care
- Showing genuine interest
- Fostering social interactions

- Inspiring patients and their families to be involved in healthcare to improve outcomes
- Being observant of mood changes and features of depression

Cultural Needs

The US is culturally diverse and promotes cultural equity in all forms of public services. For CNAs, cultural competence means awareness of the different cultural backgrounds of patients and willingness to overcome their cultural prejudices and understand diverse cultures.

Thus, while Western medicine can proclaim germs and body system malfunctions as reasons for diseases, Eastern medicine can ascribe supernatural and magical causes and suggest herbs or charms. Nurses may have to decide the safety of using these against their capacity for emotional healing.

Furthermore, Eastern medicine may lean toward holistic or natural explanations to diagnose a condition rather than a pathology. While Western medicine considers health an individual's responsibility, Eastern philosophy relies on cultural support for care. Thus, an Asian individual may refuse rehabilitative care unless their families participate.

Culturally competent nurses can interact with people from all backgrounds, appreciate unique needs and traditions, and help explain or accommodate cultural needs that can be at variance with conventional medical practice.

Sexual Needs

Sexual needs are physical intimacy of a sexual nature. It is more than acts of love-making. Touch, caress, embrace, or stroke are different ways to communicate the profound love and intimacy we crave for our emotional well-being. Diseases like diabetes and neurological disorders can decrease sexual needs. CNAs can help patients understand these needs in the following ways:

- Understanding their feelings about sexuality

- Patient entitlement to their needs and opportunities to satisfy them appropriately
- Access to privacy

However, prevent inappropriate sexual behaviors or advances, like flirting, by firmly stating your reasons. Defensive protestations by patients are unacceptable even when they are on drugs or have physical or mental disorders. Report to the immediate authorities about any undesirable sexual advances.

Spiritual Needs

Of all needs, spiritual needs are the highest and restorative. Spiritual needs, distinct from emotional and physical, are essential for feeling safe, grounded, and content. While spirituality gives hope, confidence, and the capacity to handle life changes, spiritual emptiness or distress can turn the therapeutic process futile. Illnesses and infirmity can exacerbate despite taking every measure. Patients can even lose the willpower to live.

CNAs can assist patients in reconnecting with their spiritual needs to aid healing.

- Understand patients' values.
- Listen to patients' perspectives on spirituality and spiritual needs.
- Rapport building is constructing a caring relationship with patients. They come forth with their sentiments and beliefs. They may also seek support.
- Patients must be able to practice their faith.
- Handle any religious symbol the patient uses with respect and care.

Person-Centered Care

Person-centered care considers the whole individual. The term "person" acknowledges an individual has their decision-making and participatory rights regarding self-care. A person embodies several dimensions, including intellectual, environmental, spiritual, emotional, sociocultural, and physical (CNA Certified Nursing Assistant exam Cram, 2009, 3)—all these aspects make healthcare a holistic approach. The system is conducive to improved outcomes and conforms with patients' preferences and habits. Person-centric care involves the following:

- Understand the interests, concerns, and safety of your patients.
- Communicate by adequately addressing the patients instead of using belittling terms like honey.
- Effective communication with family members helps to share information and build trust.
- Use age-appropriate words and avoid terms like potty or bib.
- Ask patient preferences for routines like time, baths, and organization of personal effects while giving ADLs.
- Respect patients' dignity and privacy while dressing and undressing them, explaining the procedures, and protecting medical information and psychological beliefs.
- Be aware of and recognize cultural differences.
- Promote self-caring abilities to uphold independence, self-control, and self-worth.

Emotional and Mental Health Needs

Mental Health Needs

Mental health needs are unique for each individual. CNAs must pay close attention to any change in the mental health status of their patients. They must identify what agitates their parents and ensure trust and care by doing their best to alleviate the concern. Thus, a basic knowledge of mental health is necessary to practice as a CNA. Some examples of mental health conditions include dementia, sundowner's syndrome, and depression.

Dementia

- Common in older patients but not a component of aging.
- Dementia has no specific symptoms.
- The most common cause of dementia is Alzheimer's disease.

- To assist patients with dementia, ensure minimal distractions, keep your directions simple, and offer limited options to prevent unrest and inconsistency.
- Report any new confusion or cognitive impairment cases to the charge nurse or doctor. Some forms of dementia (drug-induced, for instance) are reversible.

Sundowner's Syndrome

Sundowning is not a disease but a symptom collection that frequently occurs among patients with dementia in the late afternoon or evening. Sundowner's syndrome can manifest as

- Heightened confusion
- Aggressiveness
- Restlessness
- Wariness
- Being difficult

Sundowner's syndrome is common in individuals with Alzheimer's, with a prevalence of one in five cases, and requires the following interventions by a CNA:

- Restrict loud noises in the evening hours.
- Ensure well-lit rooms until bedtime.
- Promote relaxing evening activities like playing cards, music, or light reading.
- Give reassurancc.
- Avoid contradicting or arguing with patients.

Depression

- Patients in healthcare environments are at increased risk for depression due to loss of physical abilities and mental acumen.
- Encourage and listen to your patient's concerns.
- Record newly occurring or worsening depression. Symptoms of depression are

      o Exaggerated sleepiness
      o Appetite loss
      o Lack of interest in self-care or hobbies

Emotional Health

Emotional problems, unlike mental disorders, do not bear physical symptoms and are more nuanced. They require careful patient observation and discernment.

Maslow's Hierarchy of Needs

In 1943, Abraham Maslow postulated the hierarchy of needs, a set of basic needs that must be attained for fulfillment and happiness (Mcleod, 2018). He used a pyramid to describe these needs, with the most basic physiological needs forming the base. The needs are as follows from the base upward.

- Physiological needs include food, water, shelter, and clothing.
- Safety and security needs include shelter, security, control, and predictability.
- Social needs revolve around fulfilling relationships and community feelings that evoke belonging and acceptance.
- Esteem needs are feelings of self-worth, respect, and accomplishment.
- The highest need is self-actualization, which Maslow described as the full use and application of one's abilities, potentialities, skills, etc.

The importance of Maslow's theory in providing emotional healthcare is grounded on ensuring and delivering patients' physiological and safety needs before satisfying other needs.

The Five Stages of Grief

In her book, *On Death and Dying*, Elizabeth Kubler-Ross described the five stages of grief. She believed that death or a significant life change can make every one of us go through some degree of these phases. For instance, a client who became paralyzed may be in denial and angry but may never reach a state of acceptance. The stages are as follows:

- Denial: rejection of facts.
- Anger: expressions of hostility toward the bad news.
- Bargaining: negotiating to regain control over the situation. Any sentences commence with "what if" or "if only."
- Depression: expressing sorrow and withdrawal from society.
- Acceptance: although disappointed with the news, patients understand its reality and attempt to cope (Kubler-Ross, 1969).

As CNAs, you must recognize the stages of grief unique for each patient and help them come to terms with their conditions as effectively as possible.

Spiritual and Cultural Needs

Transcultural care began with Madeleine Leininger's 1950s work and her book *Culture Care Diversity and Universality: A Theory of Nursing.*

Cultures are transgenerational ideologies, attitudes, ideas, and perceptions that exclude other groups and their members. As a CNA, you must understand how culture affects patients' worldviews, beliefs, values, and experiences. It impacts an individual's health, well-being, disease, pain, and even death.

- Accept, appreciate, and embrace diversity.
- Instead of focusing on symptoms or ailments, emphasize the whole person (Leininger, 1950).
- Include cultural knowledge in therapy and alternative spiritual practices like meditation and anointing in nursing care.
- Provide solid medical advice and treatment while considering diverse cultures and concerns like traditional diets or skepticism of physicians and Western medicine.

Religious Concerns

Religion may be more entrenched and challenging to address. CNAs must respect religious views and not ignore religious concerns. Failure to uphold rules on religion and culture may result in discrimination lawsuits since religious rights and cultural perspectives are protected. To prevent this, be willing to dispel customer misunderstandings about medicine and healthcare. Show them that you work for them as a medical expert. Listen to all concerns about religion and culture and help the client overcome obstacles caused by these deeply ingrained beliefs.

Language Consideration

Using interpreters and multilingual educational materials to address customers' language challenges is acceptable. Document all procedures. The medical record should contain the client's understanding level and any translator or reading materials utilized to improve comprehension.

How well the client understands their health care condition, services, and treatments is the best approach to determine whether their linguistic requirements are satisfied.

PACE

CNAs have many tasks and details to remember. Let us understand PACE practice by considering the case of Mrs. W with dementia in a crowded nursing home set-up. She grows frustrated with care delays.

Prepare: Write down all patient duties. Sort jobs by significance and allocate time for them—schedule using the nursing care plan and a verbal report from the previous shift's caregivers or supervisor. Psychosocial care must follow five principles: safety, privacy, dignity, communication, and independence.

Assess: Prioritize which tasks? Vital sign measurements, medicine administration, meal service, and posture changes are important. The ADLs include non-specific actions like bathing and dressing. Check for preparatory needs, such as bathing. Mrs. W becomes agitated by meal service delays and rejects ADLs, prolonging the procedure. Plan around her schedule.

Carry out: Perform your vital chores and visit Mrs. W periodically to ensure she gets her care plans and attention. This job requires a smile, simple language, and encouragement.

Evaluate: Assess your performance. This step lets you know whether your intervention worked for all your patients, including Mrs. W. This strategy helps identify tasks that need more effort or a different approach.

Practice Tests

1.	What is the best response to an agitated and protesting resident?

	A. Ask the resident to calm down instead of agitating others.
	B. Provide comforting and supportive care with calmness.
	C. Report the matter to the charge nurse.
	D. Ignore the resident because he is always rude.

2.	Which is the last of the five senses to go before dying?

	A. Hearing
	B. Taste
	C. Sight
	D. Touch

3.	How would you help a resident who has just received the news of the death of a close one?

	A. Tell him that death is final.
	B. Narrate your experience with death and how you handled it.
	C. Spend time with him and empathically listen if he wants to discuss it.
	D. Encourage him to talk or think about happier things.

4.	Which is the first stage of grief by Elizabeth Kübler-Ross?

	A. Denial
	B. Anger

C. Depression

D. Acceptance

5.   How would you handle anxiety in a resident as a CNA?

A. Make the room well-lit and bright.

B. Use distractions like television.

C. Leave the spot to allow the resident to quieten down.

D. Talk calmly and show composure and assurance.

6.   A resident who tends to suffer from disorientation during evening hours is having?

A. Depression

B. Dementia

C. Sundowner's syndrome

D. Alzheimer's

7.   What is the best way to respond to a sudden sexual comment from a resident?

A. Change the course of the conversation.

B. Ignore.

C. Assert that such behavior is unacceptable.

D. Say something funny to lighten the situation.

8.   A resident is shouting and pacing the room. What should be your first action?

A. Call the change nurse.

B. Ask him to calm down.

C. Call for help.

D. Ask family members to help you quieten the resident.

9. Which of these represents cultural awareness in a healthcare facility?

    A. Cultural awareness is desirable but sometimes overlooked for cost-effectiveness.
    B. It is a must for a facility that believes in person-centered therapy.
    C. It is unfeasible in large centers with many patients.
    D. It is idealistic but impractical due to staff shortages.

10. It is time for a procedure on Mr. B. Which of the following is improper for this situation if his family wants to have some time with him for prayer?

    A. The family must leave, but Mr. B. can pray during the procedure.
    B. Give privacy to Mr. B. and his family.
    C. Inform the family you will return presently.
    D. Ask Mr. B's family if they have some queries concerning the procedure, and then allow them time for prayer.

Answers

1. B. A comforting and calming behavior is a positive response, while other options do not solve the issue and could increase agitation.

2. A. Family members and visitors may want to know that despite their inability to communicate, dying patients may still hear, which is the last sense to be lost.

3. C. Providing a caring and listening aid is all that is needed.

4. A. The first stage is generally denial for most people.

5. D. Reducing stimuli can calm anxiety.

6. C. Sundowner's syndrome occurs typically during evening hours.

7. C. Set boundaries and inform the supervisor.

8. A. The charge nurse can give medications to calm the patient.

9. B. You must be able to work with culturally diverse people.

10. A. The family should leave to commence the procedure timely, but the patient can pray.

Summary

- Psychosocial care goes beyond physical aspects and involves the individual as a whole.
- CNAs must provide emotional and basic mental health care and recognize diverse spiritual practices.
- Emotional health needs an understanding of Maslow's hierarchy of needs and the five stages of grief.
- CNAs must consider linguistic diversity.

The next chapter is on the role of nurse aide.

Chapter Four: The Role of Nurse Aide

Your role as a nurse aide will be clarified to you by your employer. Job specifications can vary according to the setting. Still, the fundamental tasks remain fixed and include the following:

- Observe the patient's rights.
- Prioritize privacy and safety.
- Provide basic and essential hygiene.
- Help residents with elimination, nutrition, and adherence to care plans.
- Execute special needs for residents with medical and mental disorders.
- Ensure smooth operations and professionalism of the work environment.

CNAs must avoid the following:

- Prescribing any medication
- Procedures requiring sterile preparations, like infusion therapy
- Prescribing treatments or home remedies
- Taking orders from resident's physicians
- Extending beyond the CNA's scope of practice
- Ignoring an order or making pretexts of not understanding an order (ask the charge nurse for clarifications, if necessary)
- Discussing medical information with residents or their family members, except colleagues who are involved with the resident's care

Overview of the Role of Nurse Aide

The chief aspects of your expected role as a nurse aide are as follows:

- Personal responsibility includes promoting healthful practices to prevent infection and harm. A clean and safe environment can check accidents and infections and reduce chances of morbidity and mortality. A clean and organized environment is also a pleasant place to work.
- Caring involves dignity and respect for your patients and your work. Avoid prejudices and welcome openness to accommodate diverse ideas and beliefs.
- Commitment to patient confidentiality, honesty, and patient care with empathy and understanding are central to the nursing profession. Report any malpractice or violation of the rules of the nursing board to the authority within a stipulated time.
- Personal health and safety, good nutrition, exercises, hobbies, and rest keep you committed and energized. Burnouts can happen in a demanding profession like nursing; preventing it will help you to remain devoted to your career.

Important Topics to Study for Nurse Aide

A nurse aide's domain of work covers the following areas:

- Knowledge of ADLs, such as feeding, bathing, toileting, and ambulating while maintaining hygiene and safety, is essential to CNAs' profession. It also includes helping with light household chores in home settings.
- Basic nursing skills: giving bedside care like ADLs, recording vital signs, and ensuring safe and efficient care are components of basic nursing skills.
- Client rights: the Patient's Bill of Rights (1973) by the American Hospital Association clarified the scope of entitlements in a healthcare setting that a CNA must be aware of.
- Communication: All communication should be simple, understandable, and direct. Address the resident by their names, and avoid using age-inappropriate or derogatory terms. Cultural competence, active listening abilities, and professional behaviors with coworkers are parts of nursing.

- Emotional and mental health requirements: CNAs care for residents' emotional and mental health, from sharing cheerful interactions to giving complex emotional support.
- Legal and ethical conduct: Unethical acts include abuse, assault, negligence, and privacy invasions. Know the nursing rules and regulations to avert wrong or unauthorized activities.
- Member of the healthcare team: As a CNA, you will be the first contact between the patient and other healthcare members. Because CNAs stay longer with their patients, they may first notice an abnormality and report it to the supervisor. It prevents costly complications.
- Restorative skills enable the residents to have self-sufficiency with most of their activities. They are also designed to prevent accidents, complications, and immobility issues.
- Spiritual and cultural requirements of healthcare settings can have varying needs, manifesting the diversity of the population in the US. CNAs have a basic understanding and appreciation of the diverse needs of residents.

Communication

Team Communication

- Communication skills with coworkers and professional respect ensure mutually trusting and collaborative effort in patient care while efficiently executing individual tasks.
- To build professional relationships, know and fulfill your assignments, document, and report consistently and responsibly. Reports must show time, observations, or changes and be factual, brief, and compact.
- Task organization according to residents' care plans and scheduling according to task and patient priorities, time, or needs for coworkers' assistance are keys to efficiency. Review residents' care plans and notes by the previous coworker. The care plan review includes

  o Name and location of the resident
  o The volume of activity
  o Transfer status

- o ADLs
- o Diet and fluid orders
- o Elimination requirements

Communication with Team Members, Residents, and Family Members

Since Florence Nightingale, nurses have relied on the concept of therapeutic communication as a vital component to encourage healing responses. As a nurse aide, you can inspire trust and sharing in your patients using the following manners of communication:

- Welcoming and introducing yourself to the patients politely.
- Asking patients warmly about their problems and responding to their reactions.
- Calmly resolving the issues and answering queries to the best of your abilities and knowledge.
- Listening nonjudgmentally to opinions.
- Respect professional boundaries.
- Understanding communication barriers and cultural needs of residents.
- Acknowledging patients' health literacy and ensuring their understanding of your communication.

Active Listening

Active listening is showing interest (eye contact) and asking for feedback (validation) from the sender of a message to understand it fully. validating a statement would be to restate it and ask whether it was what the sender meant. Competitive listening involves sharing our viewpoints rather than listening to others.

Touch

In the nursing profession, touch is a symbol showing understanding, care, and comfort. Touch should conform to patients' cultural beliefs and be respectful.

The communication symbol is often used while assessing or assisting a patient through a painful or unnerving procedure. Patients feel safe to share their thoughts and concerns.

Therapeutic Communication Techniques

The following are forms of therapeutic communication techniques in nursing.

- Silence allows patients to voice their thoughts and opinions without interference.
- Acceptance acknowledges patients' beliefs.
- Recognize healthy activities like finishing breakfast.
- Spending time is offering yourself the opportunity to build bonds.
- Open communication allows the patient to direct the flow of conversation.
- Seek elucidation for confusing statements.
- Request for time and sequence of events to better understand events.
- Observe patient behavior, appearance, etc.
- Invite descriptions of opinions.
- Encourage self-reflection in seeking solutions.
- Use constructive confrontations to break poor habits.
- Offer hope and introduce humor.

Barriers to Communication

Barriers to communication include the following:

- Jargon: Avoid medical terms, jargon, and unusual language—present facts to patients simply. Generational, geographical, or background information may affect your message.
- Attention: Task-centric rather than person-centric efforts are easy. However, following simple procedural techniques in entering a patient's room and paying complete attention to the patient are a few steps that build rapport. Regardless of your schedule, patients should feel like your priority.

- Distractions: Noise can make healthcare loud and distracting. When talking to patients, close the hallway doors, lower the TV noise, or move to a quieter space.
- Lighting: Too bright or too dim lighting can affect patient communication by interfering with their liking and comfort.
- Hearing and speech problems can affect communication. Consider using assistive devices like eyeglasses, hearing aids, whiteboards, etc.
- Language: When English is not the native tongue, seek the help of medical interpreters and provide manuals in the patient's language.
- Cultural incongruence: Social customs and emotional expression vary widely between civilizations. People from various cultures see personal space or suffering differently. Understand cultural diversity to prevent communication barriers.
- Psychological barriers: Psychological states can impact message delivery and perception. Rushing, distracting, and overloading might hinder understanding of information.
- Physiological barriers: Communicating with patients requires awareness of physiological challenges. Pain reduces a patient's ability to hear and recall.
- Physical barriers: Email and text are less successful than face-to-face communication. Misinterpreting messages is expected due to a lack of nonverbal cues. Face-to-face communication is suitable for vital information.
- Perceptive differences: Patients frequently withdraw from the discussion or treatment plan when they believe their opinions are less important. Patients can have different views and ideas. However, share information without judgment.

Hearing, Vision, and Speech Problems in Communication

Read the care plan for suggestions on preferred communication modes, like using whiteboards, pictures, etc., for communicating with patients having hearing, vision, or speech impairment. Report to the charge nurse any new changes or problems.

Impaired Hearing

Use the following methods for communication with patients having impaired hearing:

- Use assisting devices wherever applicable.
- Face the individual and draw their attention before speaking.
- Ensure minimal background noise.
- Talk slowly and distinctly without shouting.
- Use nonverbal communication.

Impaired Vision

- Identify yourself before communicating.
- Clean and store the patient's eyeglasses and help them use them throughout the day.
- Offer protective devices to reduce glare.
- Distribute instructional materials in big print.
- Read patient-relevant information.
- Provide with magnifying glasses.

Impaired Speech

Dementia, brain trauma, and stroke can reduce the capabilities of understanding and assimilating information, causing speech difficulties or aphasia.

- Individuals with expressive aphasia understand spoken communication and know their replies but cannot express themselves beyond short phrases with much effort. Instead of saying, "I want to use the bathroom," they may only be able to say, "Bathroom use."
- Individuals with receptive aphasia use long sentences without any meaning. They do not understand written and oral communication.

Use the following strategies to progress interactions in individuals with impaired speech:

- Cut off noise as much as possible and reduce emotional stress.

- Ensure the call light is reachable.
- Construct sentences having simple answers in "yes" or "no." Expressive aphasia can lead to automatic but wrong responses.
- Assess the patient's emotions due to speech impairment.
- Arrange for alternative communication modes like writing materials, flashcards, hand signs, eye blinking, or computers.
- Adjust communication style for simplicity. These are attentive listening, slow and distinct speech, facing the patient while talking, using the family's assistance to communicate effectively, etc.

Patient Rights

CNAs must be able to identify the following objectives:

- Recognize the client's right to decline therapy or procedures
- Discuss therapy alternatives or decisions with the client
- Provide client education and staff awareness about client rights and responsibilities
- Ensure client understanding of their rights
- Support client rights and requirements

The essential elements of the American Hospital Association's Bill of Rights, substituted by the Patient Care Partnership, are the following (Ivey, 2023):

- Privacy
- Confidentiality
- Esteem and dignity
- Determine their doctor(s)
- Fully learn about their medical condition and therapies
- Make independent decisions about their medical care
- Absolute exclusion of abuse and neglect
- Freedom from fear
- Emergency services
- Qualified care
- Religious and social freedom
- Having accurate bills for the care and services

- Ability to control and manage personal finances and assets
- Express their complaints and have them addressed

Right to Deny Therapy

The Patient Self Determination Act and HIPAA clarify some of the American Hospital Association's Bill of Rights (Teoli, 2022).

The Patient Self Determination Act emphasizes the individual's right to choose present and future care and treatments upon admission and initial contact.

Regardless of form, HIPAA protects clients' rights to confidentiality and privacy of medical information, including paper and computerized medical records.

Patient's Bill of Rights

The bill is a list of privileges granted to in-patients and residents in long-term care facilities. The rights include access to information, privacy, equitable and polite manners, autonomy over medical decisions, the option to reject treatment, and the right to complain.

Informed Consent

Informed consent is the patient's choice of a therapy or procedure based on their understanding of its benefits, risks, and options. Nurses must explain all nursing care and actions, except in emergencies.

There are three types of consent: implicit, explicit, or opt-out. Implicit consent, like consent for hospitalization, implies agreeing to nursing care.

Explicit consent is the direct and legal concern for acceptance or refusal of any treatment. Consent might be verbal or written. Consent for invasive procedures is usually written and recorded in the client's medical record.

Opt-out consent is passive and indirect. Patients give this consent when they do not decline therapy, which translates into not objecting to treatment or procedures.

Scope of Practice

The scope of practice for a CNA entails assignments and tasks they can do lawfully on the job. Each state's licensing board states the set of functions. CNAs risk losing their certification and legal liability for services not on the approved list.

Legal & Ethical Behavior

Be acquainted with medical ethics, standards, and the law. Knowing federal statutes on health, including the Health Insurance Portability and Accountability Act (HIPAA) is embedded in the profession.

Ethical Responsibilities

Nursing assistants should treat all clients equally and compassionately, respecting their dignity, value, and uniqueness. They should advocate for clients' rights and safety to improve health and functioning.

Avoid unethical conduct such as the following:

- Using your phone for personal purposes in patient care areas
- Neglecting call lights on duty, ignoring allocated phones, and using agency computers for personal purposes
- Ignoring clients based on race, beliefs, behavior, or other traits
- Avoiding work by resting in unoccupied patient rooms or the break room while on duty hours
- Receiving gifts or payments
- Sharing client information with those not involved in direct healthcare
- Theft of client or health care agency items

Governing Agencies

As a nursing assistant, you serve vulnerable people. Children, seniors, minorities, socially impoverished, underinsured, and some medical illnesses constitute susceptible populations. Poor health care worsens health issues in disadvantaged groups. Several regulating organizations monitor healthcare in this segment.

Centers for Medicare and Medicaid (CMS): The CMS supports health care for eligible members. Medicare covers those over 65, those with chronic disabilities, and those with kidney failure. Medicare covers hospital and nursing home care (Part A), medical appointments, services, and equipment (Part B), private company services (Part C), and prescription drugs (Part D). Medicaid is federal and state-funded health care for low-income people. Medicare and Medicaid may fund resident care depending on need.

The Centers for Disease Control (CDC) offers therapy guidelines for facilities on disease and infection control.

The Food and Drug Administration (FDA) ensures the safety of drugs, biological items, medical equipment, cosmetics, radiation-emitting products, and the food supply to safeguard public health. It controls tobacco products and provides scientific information on therapeutic products and food to maintain and promote health.

Occupational Safety and Health Administration (OSHA) maintains secure and wholesome working environments for workers by creating and implementing norms and providing training, outreach, information, and supportive programs.

Each state has a Department of Health Services (DHS) that collaborates with local counties, health care providers, and community partners. The DHS offers alcohol and drug abuse prevention, mental health, public health, disability drive, long-term care, nursing home regulation, and other services to help assist and safeguard people in the state.

Federal Health Care Acts

Federal laws shape health care in addition to government organizations. HIPAA requires national standards to secure sensitive patient health information from disclosure without permission or knowledge (sprinto, 2023). The HIPAA security regulation mandates:

- Maintain privacy, security, and accessibility of all protected health information (PHI).
- Detect and prevent identifiable information security risks.
- Prevent potential illegal uses or disclosures of PHI.
- Verify employee compliance.
- The law requires nursing assistants to keep client care information, including paperwork, care plans, and shift reports confidential.

The 1987 Omnibus Reconciliation Act (OBRA) introduced new nursing home care criteria for Medicare and Medicaid (Kelly, 1989). One necessity was nursing aide training. It provided the following mandates:

- Each state must maintain a register of new nursing aides who completed a minimum of 75 hours of training and passed a competence exam.
- Ensure improved life quality for long-term care (LTC) residents by providing patient-centered care and satisfying individual care preferences.

In 1965, politicians established the Older Americans Act (OAA) to address a shortage of community social services for seniors. The original law approved state funding for community planning and social services, research and development, and senior staff training. It also covers states' Long-Term Care (LTC) Ombudsman systems, which address health, safety, welfare, and rights issues in nursing homes, assisted living facilities, and other residential care communities (Ethical and Legal Responsibilities for the Nursing Assistants, n.d.). The OAA requirements for ombudsman programs are as follows:

- Identify, explore, and resolve resident issues.
- Inform residents about long-term services and assistance.
- Maintain regular and punctual ombudsman services for residents.

- Represent citizens before government authorities and seek administrative, legal, and other procedures to defend them.
- Research, review, and suggest resident health, safety, welfare, and rights modifications.

Liabilities

Healthcare has several liabilities. Some of them are as follows:

- Abuse is intentional physical or mental damage to a client.
- Aiding and abetting is being an "accomplice" to an offense by engaging in it or knowing about it and not reporting it. For example, you must report a CNA who had struck a confused resident to avoid liability.
- Assault and battery are legal terms. Battery is physical contact or force, whereas assault is the threat of harm.
- False confinement restricts client movement. Even keeping the doors of the room closed to prevent client movement without a doctor's orders can amount to confinement.
- Failure to protect confidential client information is a privacy invasion. HIPAA is crucial for healthcare workers. Sharing identifiable health information with an individual not directly involved in patient care may result in employment termination or legal action. HIPAA infractions, unlike assault or abuse, are not necessarily about being or doing "bad." Sharing with your relative about her friend's nursing home care progress may not seem illegal, but it may violate the friend's HIPAA rights in court.
- In healthcare, negligence or neglect implies omitting or making performance errors, causing client suffering or harm.
- Stealing is taking something without permission.

Member of the Healthcare Team

As a CNA, you must understand your roles and responsibilities as well as those of others involved in patient care. It helps you know whom you should contact in case of client need, besides your obligations.

The core team is formed by the physician in charge of the patient's care, the nursing staff (including the licensed nurse, medical aides, and CNAs), and the patient's family. The physical therapist, social worker, chaplain, or spiritual counselor all play important roles in the patient's recovery. You may have additional responsibilities depending on the healthcare setting.

CNA's Role

CNAs' roles are crucial to healthcare setups. You may spend the most time with the client. Hence, you are likely to notice changes before other healthcare professionals. Provide direct care, ensure the client's comfort, safety, and welfare, and assist them in achieving their health objectives.

ADLs

ADLs include bathing, dressing, eating, managing hygiene and toileting, positioning, transferring, ambulating, and communicating, and are the main objectives.

As a CNA, you help patients in being comfortable physically and emotionally. Maintaining a clean and pleasant atmosphere enhances safety and therapeutic recovery.

Safety

CNAs are directly responsible for ensuring resident safety. Following procedural guidelines, alertness, and promptness in reporting minor or marked changes in the client's status to supervisors provides resident safety. Avoid circumstances that might jeopardize residents or lead to negligence charges. Address client distress promptly responding to the call light.

Practice infection control to keep the surroundings clean—body fluids are contaminated. Handwashing before and after care and using gloves for procedures that require exposure to body fluids, such as cleaning a urine drainage bag are effective.

Evaluation and Assistance

Document any changes in appearance, attitude, disposition, behavior, vitality, or complaints. Observe bruising, pain, unpleasant smells, and patient complaints objectively to avoid bias.

Inform the charge nurse of any changes, concerns, or abnormalities. Report the vital signs that are crucial for the whole healthcare team in patient management. These are as follows:

- Pulse
- Temperature
- Blood pressure
- Respiration
- Weight
- Food and beverage consumption
- Elimination habits

When the licensed nurse is administering treatments or procedures, the CNA may help. Learn the legal limits of the processes you can (cannot refuse or excuse) or cannot (may refuse) participate.

Professional and Professionalism

Professional is anything concerned with one's profession or occupation. Professionalism is the manner in which individuals carry themselves while on the job, including the way they talk, share information, carry out tasks, follow orders, and dress.

Professionalism embodies compassion (being kind and caring), empathy (the ability to identify others' pain), and sympathy (sharing others' feelings and difficulties). Other features are tactfulness (consideration and appropriateness of interactions) and conscientiousness (integrity and reliability).

The professional conduct of CNAs include

- Optimistic attitude
- Being on time
- Performing assigned tasks only
- Not talking about personal matters
- Maintaining patient confidentiality
- Addressing residents by proper names with courtesy and politeness
- Listening
- Avoiding abuse or neglect
- Observing, documenting, and prompt reporting of any patient changes to supervisors.

Transparency

For healthcare practitioners, transparency is sharing as much information as possible for safe treatment. It means having and sharing all information pertaining to optimal patient care and builds trust.

PACE

Let us consider the example of Mrs. V, a CNA, regarding how she manages patient care in her busy schedule ethically and legally by adhering to the PACE strategy.

The strategy emphasizes the necessity to prepare for all contingencies that are expected to crop up during patient care. Mrs. V responds to the sudden scream from the corridor while she bathes a resident. Which step must she prepare before she attends to the commotion? And should she attend to the noise at all?

Ensuring patient safety is critical to nursing. CNAs should attend to disturbances to check for assistance needs. Before doing so, they must ensure the safety of their patients. They should return to their station as quickly as possible.

Maintaining high legal and ethical practice standards requires preparation (mental and physical), assessment of the situation according to all available information and making decisions objectively and ethically, execution according to task priority, and evaluation of all your tasks per standards.

Thus, if a resident is shaky, your instinctual preparation would tell you to do a blood sugar test first. The test can help you to assess the condition. If the results are low, you may give the resident glucose, which is task execution per your assessment to the best of your knowledge and ability. Afterward, evaluate if the resident's symptoms have gone.

Questions

1. A care plan mentions administering a medication TID. How many times should the medicine be given?

    A. Twice daily.
    B. Thrice daily.
    C. Once daily.
    D. Do not give the medicine.

2. Listening is sometimes the best therapy; which is the best way to listen?

    A. Ask direct questions to guide the conversation.
    B. Discuss your experience on the matter.
    C. Face the resident and speak when appropriate.
    D. Talk to the resident while working.

3. Any procedure must follow steps from beginning to finish. Which of these is the initial step?

    A. Record the date.
    B. Verify resident identification.
    C. Ensure privacy.
    D. Document your task.

4. Which communication strategy should be best for a resident with complete hearing impairment?

    A. Phone with amplifiers.
    B. Use a loud voice.
    C. Use an audible alarm.
    D. Use a laptop or pen and paper.

5. Which of these is not included in medical documentation?

    A. Author identification.
    B. Timing the tasks.
    C. Avoid spelling mistakes.
    D. Use pencils to erase any mistakes made.

6. For a patient undergoing surgery the next day, which of these abbreviations suggests "nothing orally."

    A. NPO
    B. NO
    C. NOT
    D. NPA

7. Which of the following is not negligence?

    A. Not remaining on the floor after signing in
    B. Keeping a jutted overhead tray open
    C. Not shifting an immobile resident enough to prevent bed sores
    D. Forgetting to provide enough drinking water punctually

8. Administering the wrong medication to a resident is an example of ___.

    A. Malpractice
    B. Assault
    C. Battery
    D. Negligence

9. Verbally threatening a resident is an example of ___.

    A. Maligning
    B. Assault
    C. Battery
    D. Slander

10. What should be the first action to respond to a contained fire in a resident's room?

    A. Ensure patient safety.
    B. Pull the fire alarm.
    C. Use the fire extinguisher
    D. Shout for assistance.

Answers

1. B. TID means thrice daily.

2. C. Facing and making eye contact are examples of active listening.

3. B. Checking residents' identification is the first step.

4. D. Visual communication is most helpful since the resident can read and understand)

5. D. Legal documents are final and cannot be erased)

6. A. NPO means nothing per mouth. The patient will have no food or beverage.

7. A. You may need to move across the facility for various assignments. Task completion ethically and safely is a priority.

8. A. Failure to perform medical duties causing patient harm is malpractice.

9. B. Assault is a threat, while battery is physical harm. Maligning and slander are making defamatory statements.

10. A. Since the fire is contained, the first step would be to shift patients from its reach to protect them from fire-related injuries and harm. Other measures should follow this procedure.

Summary

- CNA's responsibility includes promoting healthful practices to prevent infection and harm.
- All communication should be simple, understandable, and direct. Maintain cultural competence and use patient-friendly methods to communicate.
- CNAs must understand patient rights.
- Remain within your professional obligations. Identify supervising authority and delegating principles for your facility.
- Maintain professionalism of practice.

In the next chapter, you will learn about skills tests and how to prepare for them.

Chapter Five: Skills Test Preparation

Your domain skills make you a vital communication link between patients and their medical teams; thus, you must utilize precise medical language when relaying patient information to physicians and collaborating with other healthcare team members. Professional conduct and professionalism is essential to honor your practice and maintain legal boundaries.

Your bedside manner may make or break a patient's experience. Compassion and understanding can heal wounds that medicines can't mitigate.

For all your preparations, you may never know what to expect from day to day. Because of nationwide CNA shortages, CNAs may have to work overtime, on weekends, or on a different shift than planned.

But you will only be effective as a CNA if you know proper technical skills. It is the area where exercising the PACE method is most strategic.

Explanation of Skills Demonstration Section of the Test

For the CNA test, the purpose of the skills test is to test your ability to perform well in a real-world caring setting. The testing area will appear like a standard office. It comes fully stocked with everything you need to carry out your duties. A Nurse Aide Evaluator will give you the test. The evaluator will apprise you of the necessary equipment and answer any questions you may have before the actual skills exam starts.

What You May Expect

A volunteer will portray the role of an older client. You would talk to them like a nurse aide client while doing the tasks. Speaking with the client is part of caring and will help you relax while doing the skills. The prerequisites for a test include the following criteria:

- You will not receive any assistance.
- The communication language is English.

Volunteering to be a patient for the skills test of another nurse aide candidate is a requirement. The evaluator will provide verbal instructions on how to play the client's role.

Dress Code

The dress code for the skills test includes flat, slip-on, non-skid shoes, a loose-fitting blouse with short sleeves that you can roll up to the shoulder, or a tank top and baggy trousers that you can similarly roll up. On top of this attire, you must don a gown before entering.

If you have any known allergies, such as to foods, latex, soaps, or lotions, inform the examiner before the test begins. Also, notify the evaluator of any range-of-motion restrictions at this time. Visiting the testing facility with cuts, scrapes, or other open wounds is not advisable. Candidates with open cuts or sores should postpone their skills test until their skin has completely healed.

What are the Skills?

The Skills Evaluation requires you to show items enlisted in the NNAAP Skills List. Each skill has sequentially arranged steps. A highlighted step is the Critical Element step for that skill. To pass the skill, you must complete Critical Element Steps accurately. You will fail the skill if you skip or perform a Critical Element Step erroneously.

Successfully completing the Critical Element of a skill test does not guarantee passing the test. Each skill has a passing score that you may obtain by executing several steps correctly. The Nurse Aide Evaluator will provide you with an instruction card before the beginning of the test. It contains details of the five (5) skills they have chosen for you to exhibit. The handwashing skill is compulsory. Doing the skills in sequence on the instruction card. One of the four randomly chosen skills will be a measurement skill. Disinfect your hands before moving from demonstrating skills on subjects to inanimate client skills.

Acing the Skills Test

Ace the skill tests with an understanding of the following topics:

Opening Procedure

It includes the following steps:

- Knock on the door
- Introduce yourself
- Explain the procedure
- Wash your hands
- Verify resident identity
- Adjust and lock the bed

- Close curtains
- Wear the gloves
- Start the procedure

Closing Procedure

- Remove used gloves
- Wash hands
- Give a call light to the resident
- Lower the bed all the way
- Open curtains
- Wash hands
- Document

Do's and Don'ts

The do's list is sharp and precise. Start the test with opening procedures, read the care plan thoroughly, and prepare to follow it to the T. If you forget a step, tell the patient, and correct it promptly. This way, the evaluator understands you know you missed a step and when to do it. Review the the care plan. Redoing the skill can shorten your time.

Do not rush through the steps or recite them openly to avoid others learning from your efforts.

Step-by-Step Checklist of 23 Skills

Practice the skills in the same sequence of steps as mentioned. The bold numbers are the Critical Elements. The best way to carry out the steps is to remember the PACE method or prepare the setting, assess the patient, task, and situation, carry out the procedure you have chalked in your mind, and evaluate your performance.

Skill 1: Handwashing

1. Address and introduce yourself to the patient by name.
2. Turn on the sink water.
3. Thoroughly wet hands and wrists.
4. Use soap on your hands.
5. **Lather, applying friction to wrists, hands, and fingers for 20 seconds, keeping hands below elbows and fingertips down.**
6. Clean nails by rubbing fingers against opposite palms.
7. **Rinse wrists, hands, and fingers, ensuring hands are below elbows and fingertips are down.**
8. Dry fingers, hands, and wrists using clean, dry paper towels, then discard them in the garbage bin.
9. Utilize clean, dry paper towels to turn off the faucet and discard them in the garbage bin using knee/foot control.
10. Never touch the inner side of the sink.

Skill 2: Apply One-Knee High Elastic Stocking

1. Explain the procedure, providing clear, slow, and straightforward instructions, aiming for face-to-face contact wherever feasible.
2. Pull curtains, screens, and doors to give privacy.
3. The client lies supine on the bed during stocking.
4. Turn the stocking inside-out, at least to the heel.
5. Place the stocking's foot over the toes, foot, and heel.
6. Pull the stocking top over the foot, heel, and leg.
7. Move the foot and leg gently and naturally, avoiding force and joint overextension.
8. **Complete operation with no twists or wrinkles, heel over heel, toe opening over or under the toe, and mention using wrinkle-free stockings if using a mannequin.**
9. The bed is low, and the signaling device is accessible.
10. Wash hands after skill.

Skill 3: Using Transfer Belts to Ambulate Patients

1. Explain the procedure.
2. Ensure privacy.
3. **Ensure the patient is wearing non-skid footwear.**
4. Ensure the bed is at a secure level.
5. Ensure the bed wheels are locked.
6. **Help the patient sit on the bed with their feet flat.**
7. Tie the transfer belt securely around the waist over clothing or gown.

Give instructions to help the patient stand, including predetermined cues to alert the patient to start standing.

8. Carry out steps 1–7 before helping the patient to stand.
9. Stand facing the client, positioning yourself for the patient and your own safety during ambulation.
10. Give the cue (counting to three) to alert the patient to start standing. On the signal, help the client stand slowly by holding the transfer belt on its sides with an upward grasp; maintain patient stability by positioning knee to knee or toe to toe with them.
11. Holding onto the belt, walk slightly behind and to one side of the patient, covering a ten-foot distance.
12. Help the patient back in bed and remove the transfer belt.
13. Ensure the signaling device is within patient reach and the bed is low.
14. Wash hands.

Skill 4: Using Bedpan

1. Explain the procedure.
2. Ensure privacy.
3. Lower the head-end of the bed.
4. Wear clean gloves before placing the bedpan under the patient.

Steps 1–4 are before giving the bedpan.

5. Position the bedpan correctly under the buttocks.

6. Remove and dispose of the gloves into the waste container without contaminating yourself. Wash hands.
7. Raise the head-end of the bed after steps 5–6.
8. Keep toilet tissue within reach.
9. The hand wipe should be within reach; instruct the patient to clean their hands after finishing.
10. Ensure the availability of a signaling device; ask the patient to signal when finished.
11. Wear clean gloves before removing the bedpan.
12. Lower the head-end of the bed before removing the bedpan.
13. Ensure covering the patient except while placing or removing the bedpan.
14. Empty the bedpan and rinse, pouring the rinse into the toilet.
15. Keep the bedpan in a designated place for dirty supplies.
16. Remove and dispose of gloves into a waste container without self-contamination. Wash hands.
17. Ensure the availability of the signaling device and lowered bed position.

Skill 5: Cleaning Upper or Lower Dentures

1. Wear clean gloves.
2. Line the sink bottom and fill it partly with water. Hold the denture over the sink.
3. Rinse the denture at a moderate temperature before brushing it.
4. Apply denture toothpaste to a toothbrush.
5. Brush both surfaces.
6. Rinse in moderate-temperature running water.
7. Rinse the denture cup and lid.
8. Place the denture in a denture cup with moderate-temperature water or solution and cover the top.
9. Rinse the toothbrush and place it in the designated basin or container.
10. Maintain a clean procedure with toothbrush and denture positionings.
11. Remove the sink liner or drain it appropriately, discarding the material.
12. Remove and dispose of gloves into a waste container without self-contamination. Wash hands.

Skill 6: Count and Record Radial Pulse

1. Explain the procedure.
2. Position your fingertips on the notch of the patient's wrist on the thumb side. Feel the radial pulse.
3. Count the beats for one minute.
4. Make the signal device available.
5. Wash hands before recording.
6. **Record reading within plus or minus four beats of the test taker's reading.**

Skill 7: Count and Record Respiration

1. Explain the procedure.
2. Count respirations for one minute.
3. Keep the signaling device at hand.
4. Wash hands before recording.
5. **Record reading within plus or minus two breaths of the test taker's reading.**

Skill 8: Donning and Doffing PPE

1. Lift the gown and unfold it.
2. Hold the gown's back open and pass both arms through each sleeve.
3. Fasten the neck cords.
4. Fasten the back ties, ensuring your back clothing is covered maximally by the gown.
5. Wear gloves.
6. The cuffs of the gloves must overlap the folds of the gown.
7. **Before doffing the gown, remove one glove by grasping it at the palm with the other gloved hand.**
8. **Slip your fingers of the ungloved hand underneath the cuff of the other glove at the wrist and remove this glove by turning it inside out.**
9. Dispose of gloves into a designated waste container without self-contamination.
10. Unfasten the gown at the waist and neck.

11. Remove the gown without touching its outer surface.
12. While removing the gown, hold it away from the body without touching the floor. Turn the gown inward and keep it inside out.
13. Discard the gown into a designated waste container without self-contamination.
14. Wash hands.

Skill 9: Dress the Patient with an Affected (Right) Arm

1. Explain the procedure.
2. Provide privacy.
3. Ask the patient's preference for a dress.
4. Keep the chest covered to prevent overexposure.
5. Remove the gown from the unaffected (strong) side and then from the affected (weak) arm.
6. Discard the gown in a soiled linen container before dressing the patient.
7. **Help the patient put the affected arm through the sleeve of the dress before passing the sleeve through the unaffected side.**
8. While dressing, move the body gently and naturally, avoiding jerks and overstretching of arms and joints.
9. Finish dressing.
10. Ensure the bed is low and the signaling devise is available.
11. Wash hands.

Skill 10: Feeding Patients Who Cannot Feed Self

1. Explain the procedure.
2. Read the name card and ask the patient to state their name before starting the procedure.
3. **Ensure the patient is upright ($\angle 75° – \angle 90°$).**
4. Place the food tray in the patient's line of vision.
5. Clean the patient's hands before feeding them.
6. Sit on a chair facing the patient.
7. Describe the foods and beverages to the patient.
8. Ask what the patient would like to eat first.

9. Offer one bite of each food type with a spoon, telling the patient the content of each spoonful.
10. Offer beverages at least once during meals.
11. Enquire the patient's readiness before passing them the next helping of food or drink.
12. Clean the patient's hands and mouth after the meal.
13. Remove the food tray.
14. Position the patient upright ($\angle 75° - \angle 90°$) with a signaling device at hand.
15. Wash hands.

Skill 11: Giving Modified Bath (Face and One Arm, Hand and Underarm)

1. Explain the procedure.
2. Provide privacy.
3. Cover the patient's chest and lower body while removing the gown into a soiled linen container.
4. Check water temperature for safety and comfort and seek patient's confirmation.
5. Wear clean gloves before bathing.
6. **Start with washing the eyes with a wet washcloth (no soap). Each stroke should be with a different area of the washcloth. Wash the eyes from the inner to the outer side before proceeding to the face.**
7. Dry the face with a dry cloth towel or a washcloth.
8. Expose one arm and place a cloth towel underneath it.
9. Apply soap to a wet washcloth.
10. Wash fingers, including fingernails, hand, arm, and underarm, covering the rest of the body.
11. Rinse and dry fingers and the hand, arm, and underarm.
12. Throughout the procedures, move the body gently and naturally, avoiding jerks and overstretching of arms and joints.
13. Put a clean gown on the patient.
14. Empty, rinse, and dry the basin.
15. Keep the basin in the ear-marked dirty supply zone.
16. Discard the linen into the soiled linen container.
17. Avoid contact between your dress and the used linens.

18. Remove and discard gloves into a waste container without self-contamination. Wash hands.
19. Ensure the bed is low and the availability of the signaling device.

Skill 12: Measure and Record Electronic Blood Pressure

1. Explain the procedure.
2. Provide privacy.
3. Position the patient comfortably, sitting or lying.
4. The patient's arm is positioned at the heart level with palm facing up and upper arm exposed.
5. Choose the appropriate cuff size.
6. At the bend of the elbow joint, feel for the brachial artery pulsations on the inner side of the arm.
7. Tie the cuff on the upper arm snugly with the sensor or arrow over the brachial artery.
8. Turn on the machine and ensure its functioning. Select the specific setting for the age of the patient if the machine has different settings for age.
9. Press the start button. If the cuff inflates to more than 200 mm Hg, stop the machine and use the cuff on the other side.
10. Wait until the readings appear on the screen and the cuff deflates. Remove the cuff.
11. Ensure signaling device availability.
12. Wash hands.
13. **Record systolic and diastolic pressures exactly as displayed on the digital screen after obtaining results using the BP cuff.**

Skill 13: Measure and Record Urinary Output

1. Wear clean gloves before handling the bedpan.
2. Pour its content into a measuring container, taking care not to spill urine outside.
3. Rinse the bedpan and empty the rinse into the toilet.
4. Keep the container flat and measure the urine quantity at eye level. If the volume is between two measuring lines, round up to the nearest 25 ml/cc.

5. Empty the measuring container in the toilet after measuring the urine volume.
6. Rinse the container and drain the rinse into the toilet.
7. Before recording the urine output, remove and discard the gloves in a waste container and wash your hands.
8. **Record the urine volume within plus or minus 25 ml/cc of the evaluator's recording.**

Skill 14: Measure and Record the Weight of Ambulatory Patient

1. Explain the procedure.
2. Ensure the patient is wearing non-skid shoes before taking their weight.
3. Before the process, set the weighing scale to zero.
4. Ask the patient to stand in the center of the scale and look up as you take the weight.
5. Ask the patient to get down from the scale.
6. Wash hands.
7. **Record the weight as shown in the indicator on the scale. The weight must be within plus or minus 2 lbs or 0.9 kg of the assessor's reading.**

Skill 15: Perform Modified Passive Range of Motion (PROM) for One Knee and One Ankle

1. Explain the procedure.
2. Provide patient privacy.
3. The patient must be supine on the bed. Instruct the patient to tell if they feel pain during the exercise.
4. Support the exercising leg at the knee and ankle and bend the knee. Then, return the leg to the normal position (flexion and extension). Repeat PROM at least thrice unless the patient complains of pain. Move the joints slowly and gently through their range of motion and discontinue whenever the patient complains of pain.
5. **Support the foot and ankle close to the bed, and push or pull the foot upward, toes pointing toward the ceiling (dorsiflexion). Then, push or**

pull the foot down, toes pointing downward (plantar flexion). Repeat the ROM at least thrice unless the patient complains of pain. Move the joints slowly and carefully through the ranges of motion and discontinue if the patient complains of pain.

6. Keep the signaling device within the reach of the patient and the bed low.
7. Wash hands.

Skill 16: Perform Modified Passive Range of Motion (PROM) for One Shoulder

1. Explain the procedure.
2. Provide patient privacy.
3. The patient must be supine on the bed. Ask them to inform you if they experience pain during the exercise.
4. **Support the arm at the elbow and the wrist, lift the patient's arm straight up, and then move it alongside the ear toward the head. Return the arm down at the body's side (flexion/extension). Repeat the ROM thrice unless the patient voices pain. Move the joints slowly and carefully through the ranges of motion and stop the exercise if the patient complains of pain.**
5. **Support the patient's arm at the elbow and at the wrist and move the straightened arm away from the body's side to shoulder level and return to the side of the body (abduction/adduction). Carry out the exercise at least three times carefully and slowly, and discontinue anytime the patient voices pain.**
6. Keep the signaling device within the reach of the patient and the bed low.
7. Wash hands.

Skill 17: Turning the Patient on Their Side

1. Explain the procedure.
2. Provide patient privacy.
3. Lower the head-end of the bed before turning the patient.
4. Raise the bedrail on the side where you are turning the patient.
5. Help the patient to roll slowly on the side toward the raised side rail.

6. Place a pillow or adjust one under the patient's head for support.
7. Reposition the patient's arm and shoulder to ensure they are not lying on their arm.
8. Support the top arm with a supporting device.
9. Position a supporting device behind the patient's back.
10. Position a supporting device between the legs, flexing the top knee. Support the knee and the ankle.
11. Keep the signaling device within the reach of the patient and the bed low.
12. Wash hands.

Skill 18: Provide Catheter Care for Females

1. Explains procedure
2. Provide patient privacy.
3. Check the water temperature for safety and comfort and ask the patient to verify it before washing.
4. Wear clean gloves.
5. Place linen protector under perineal area, including buttocks.
6. Expose the region surrounding the catheter, taking care to uncover the patient's body between hip and knee only.

Do the steps 1–6 before washing.

7. Apply soap to a wet washcloth.
8. **While holding the catheter at the meatus without tugging, clean at least four inches of the catheter from the meatus, moving in only one direction away from the meatus. Use a clean position of the washcloth for each stroke.**
9. **While you hold the catheter at the meatus without tugging, rinse at least four inches from the meatus, moving in only one direction: away from the meatus. Use a clean position of the washcloth for each stroke.**
10. While you hold the catheter at the meatus without tugging, dry at least four inches of the catheter from the meatus, moving in only one direction: away from the meatus. Use a dry towel cloth or washcloth.
11. Empty the basin, rinse it, and then dry it.
12. Keep the basin in the designated dirty container zone.

13. Discard used linen into a soiled linen container and dispose of the linen protector properly.
14. Ensure no contact between your clothing and the soiled linen.
15. Remove and discard gloves into a waste container, not contaminating yourself. Wash hands.
16. Keep the signaling device within patient reach and the bed position low.

Skill 19: Provide Foot Care on One Foot

1. Explain the procedure.
2. Secure patient privacy.
3. Check water temperature for safety and comfort, and ask the patient to verify their comfort level.
4. Keep the basin comfortable for the patient and on a protective barrier.

Steps 1–5 are before washing and include preparatory and assessment steps before carrying out the procedure on the patient.

1. Wear clean gloves.
2. Place the patient's foot in the water.
3. Apply soap to a wet washcloth.
4. Lift the foot from water and wash the foot, including the spaces between toes.
5. Rinse the foot, including the spaces between the toes.
6. Dry the foot and the spaces between the toes.
7. Apply lotion to the top and bottom of the foot. Do not apply lotion in the spaces between the toes. Remove excess lotion with a towel or a washcloth.
8. Support the foot and ankle throughout the procedure.
9. Empty, rinse, and dry the basin.
10. Keep the basin in the earmarked dirty supply area.
11. Discard used linen into a soiled linen container.
12. Remove and discard gloves into a waste container, taking care not to contaminate yourself. Wash hands.
13. Keep the signaling device within patient reach and the bed position low.

Skill 20: Give Mouth Care

1. Explain the procedure.
2. Secure patient privacy.
3. The patient must be sitting upright before you give them mouth care ($\angle 75° - \angle 90°$).
4. Wear clean gloves before cleaning the mouth.
5. Place a cloth towel across the patient's chest before giving mouth care.
6. Secure the water cup, and moisten a toothbrush.
7. Apply toothpaste to a wet toothbrush before cleaning the mouth.
8. **Clean the patient's mouth, including their tongue and both surfaces of teeth. Make gentle motions.**
9. Place the toothbrush, maintaining hygienic techniques.
10. Wipe the mouth and remove the clothing protector.
11. Discard used linen into the container for soiled linen.
12. Rinse the toothbrush and empty, rinse, and dry the basin.
13. Remove and discard the gloves, taking care to avoid self-contamination. Wash hands.
14. Keep the signaling device at hand and the bed low.

Skill 21: Give Perineal Care (Peri-Care) for Female

1. Explain the procedure.
2. Provide patient privacy.
3. Check the water temperature for safety and comfort, and ask the patient to verify before washing.
4. Wear clean gloves.
5. Palace a pad or linen protector under the perineal area, including the buttocks.
6. Expose the perineal area, only uncovering the area between hips and knees.
7. Apply soap to a wet washcloth.
8. **Wash the genital area, moving from front to back; use a clean portion of the washcloth for each stroke you apply.**
9. **Taking a clean washcloth, rinse soap from the genital area. Apply the strokes from front to back. Use a clean portion of the washcloth for each stroke.**

10. Dry the genital region using a dry washcloth or towel. Move from front to back.
11. Turn the patient to their side after washing the genital region, and wash the rectal area from front to back with a clean part of the washcloth for every stroke.
12. Use a clean washcloth, and rinse soap from the rectal area, moving from front to back. Use a clean area of the washcloth for each stroke.
13. Dry the rectal area, moving from front to back, with a dry cloth towel or washcloth.
14. Reposition the patient.
15. Empty, rinse, and dry the basin.
16. Place the basin in the earmarked area for dirty supplies.
17. Discard used linen into a soiled linen container and linen protector properly.
18. Avoid contact between your clothing and used linen.
19. Remove and discard gloves onto a waste container without self-contamination. Wash hands.
20. Ensure the availability of the signaling device and keep the bed low.

Skill 22: Transfer the Patient from the Bed to the Wheelchair Using the Transfer Belt

1. Explain the procedure.
2. Provide patient privacy.
3. Position the wheelchair alongside the bed, at the head of the bed facing the foot, or at the foot of the bed facing the head.
4. Fold or remove the footrests.
5. **Lock the wheels on the wheelchair.**
6. Ensure the bed is at a safe height.
7. Check and lock the bed wheels.
8. **Assist the patient to a sitting posture with their feet resting on the floor.**
9. Ensure the patient has their shoes on.
10. Apply the transfer belt securely at the waist over the gown or clothing.
11. Instruct the patient on the transfer procedure you will follow, including a predetermined signal to alert the time to start to stand.

Steps 3–11 are before assisting the patient to stand.

1. Stand facing the patient to ensure your and the patient's safety during transfer. Alert the patient to begin standing by counting three or any other predetermined signal.
2. Assist the patient in standing on the signal by holding the transfer belt on both sides with your hands upward. Your movements must be slow and steady. Provide stability to the posture by standing knee to knee or toe to toe with the patient.
3. Help the patient turn to stand in front of the wheelchair with the back of their legs pressing the wheelchair.
4. Gradually lower the patient to the wheelchair.
5. Position the patient with hips next to the back of the wheelchair and remove the transfer belt.
6. Position the patient's feet on the footrests.
7. Keep the signaling device at hand.
8. Wash hands.

Skill 23: Measure and Record Manual Blood Pressure (BP)

This is a state-specific test and not replaced by a skill test to record electronic BP.

1. Explain the procedure.
2. Wipe the bell or diaphragm of the stethoscope with alcohol before using it.
3. Position the patient's arm with the palm upward and expose the upper arm.
4. Feel brachial artery pulsations on the inner side of the arm at the bend of the elbow joint.
5. Tie the BP cuff firmly around the upper arm with the sensor or arrow over the brachial artery site.
6. Put the stethoscope's earpieces inside your ears and the stethoscope bell over the brachial artery region.
7. Inflate the cuff between 160 mmHg–180 mmHg. Deflate the cuff completely upon immediately hearing arterial pulsations. Inflate the cuff not exceeding 200 mmHg.
8. Deflate the cuff slowly and note the first sound (systolic BP) and the last (diastolic BP). Round measurements, if required, UP to the closest two mmHg.

9. Remove the cuff.
10. Keep the signaling device within reach.
11. Wash hands before recording.
12. **After getting a BP reading with a BP cuff and stethoscope, record systolic and diastolic pressures within plus or minus eight mmHg of the assessor's recordings.**

For all skills, explain the procedures slowly, clearly, and directly, facing the patient whenever possible. Maintain patient privacy during the procedure using a curtain, screen, or closing the door.

A clinical skills test evaluates indirect care skills, abbreviated as IC. It includes greeting the patient by using their first names and introducing yourself; explaining the procedure before beginning the procedure and during it; asking about the patient's preferences; observing the patient's safety, rights, and dignity during care; and asking about their comfort or needs before or during care. Ensure IC before and during all care skills.

PACE Method in Skills Test

Nowhere is the PACE method better applied than in the clinical skills demonstration component of the CNA test. You are observed, assessed, and scored on every aspect of the procedures. Handwashing and IC skills are mandatory and are scored for each test.

Preparation also means physical preparation. Most of the tests have several steps before you actually begin the procedure. It will require assembling the correct materials that you need for each test on your list.

Assessment is about checking the instructions, patient condition, and the situation. Patient and self-safety are of prime concern. For bathing, for instance, you will assess the water temperature and seek patient verification.

Carrying out the procedure requires diligence and deftness. For handwashing, for instance, you will be tested on whether you used friction to spread soap and create lather to clean for at least 20 seconds the front and back of hands, between fingers, around cuticles, under nails, and wrists.

Finally, evaluation means checking whether you performed all the steps correctly. The best way to ensure this is to see if the patient is satisfied and comfortable.

Skills Practice

Here are some tips to ace the CNA skills test:

1. Daily practicing the clinical procedures on a family member or a friend will help you to sharpen your practice, follow the PACE method closely, and make them your habits that you regularly perform.
2. Dress professionally.
3. The evaluator needs to see how concerned you are with patient safety. Cover the patient during personal care, raise the bedrails to secure the patient, and use transfer belts properly. Patient safety also means properly donning and disposing of PPEs.
4. Ensure you understand the scenario of a skill test well. You can ask clarifying questions before you begin, but not once you start.
5. Respond to your mistake promptly and seek to repeat the steps. Prompt self-evaluation and redressal help you to gain favorable points from the evaluator.
6. Practice safe body mechanics by bending at the knees, positioning yourself comfortably, and lifting after securing proper foot support.
7. Ensure all tools are cleaned before and after you use them. These are a bell of a stethoscope, thermometers, or BP cuffs. Wipe them with alcohol before replacing them in their boxes. Rinse and air dry wash basins and discard used linens into the designated container without contaminating your clothes.
8. Handwashing before and after a procedure is necessary, and forgetting it can fail you in the performance test. Wash your hands when in doubt.
9. Practice giving care with respect. Although you will not test your skills on a real patient, your performance should exhibit all the aspects of hospitality. Greet, explain the procedure, provide privacy, and ask about preferences, even if it is a model.

10. Practice extensively to reduce any performance-related anxiety.
11. Check the correct methods for enacting the skills on YouTube by typing in CNA skills or the name of a particular skill.
12. Headmaster.com and Prometric provide a candidate handbook with step-by-step instructions on the skills. They familiarize you with the elements the evaluators will assess (Generic Nurse Aide Clinical Skills Checklist, n.d.).
13. Make big flashcards, writing each step in bold on one side and the name of the skill on the other. Review them periodically until you learn them by heart.
14. Testing techniques can vary among states. Check the specifications for your state on state websites (Ball, 2021).

Summary

- The Skills Evaluation includes items enlisted in the NNAAP Skills List.
- To pass the skill, you must complete Critical Element Steps accurately.
- Each skill has a passing score you obtain by executing several steps correctly.
- Practice each skill extensively to reduce any performance-related anxiety.

The next chapter is on practice tests that test your CNA knowledge.

Part 2: Practice Tests

Chapter Six: Practice Test 1

This chapter is the first of a series of practice runs on the CNA test. The entire chapter consists of several sections with questions on each of them. In total, there are 60 questions. Time your test similarly to complete the practice test. The answer key and the explanation are in the appendix section.

1.   In which situations should a resident use a soft Toothette oral swab?

    A. When the resident has convulsions.
    B. When the resident has a toothache.
    C. A resident using dentures.
    D. An unconscious resident while receiving mouth care.

2.   A patient recovering from a stroke has weakness on his left side. While dressing this patient, from which side will you approach?

    A. From the left side
    B. From his front
    C. From his right side
    D. From his back

3.   Which of the following procedures is not favorable for providing hygienic care?

    A. Dry the patient's skin after washing to prevent contagion.
    B. Encourage resident participation.

C. Examine the skin for injuries or bruises before giving a bath.

D. Apply lotion generously with additional coverage between digits.

4. A CNA is assisting a patient with quadriplegia to eat. Which of the following actions is not encouraged?

A. Sit at the patient's eye level.

B. Offer the patient small bites and give them time to chew and swallow.

C. Offer beverages once the entire meal is finished.

D. Talk to the patient about the foods and drinks on the tray.

5. Which of the following is NOT a familiar problem residents encounter in a healthcare facility?

A. Not being reminded about mealtimes

B. Loss of ability to use silverware

C. Chewing problems

D. Decreased response to thirst and hunger

6. Which of the following is an intake and output problem that a nurse aide must report to the charge nurse?

A. The resident wants a bedpan.

B. Urine output in eight hours is 700 cc.

C. The resident has not voided in eight hours.

D. The resident states as not being hungry.

7. What should be the patient's position to receive an enema?

A. Prone

B. Supine

C. Fowler's

D. Left Sim's

8. To clean a female patient's perineum, a CNA must use which of the following techniques?

A. Clean from back to front.

    B. Clean from front to back.

    C. Use a disinfectant.

    D. Avoid soap.

9. Morning care, also known as AM care, is given for which of the following purposes?

    A. It reduces harmful microbes.

    B. It improves appearance.

    C. It promotes patient well-being.

    D. All of the above.

10. You notice red marks on a resident's back and buttocks. What should be your action?

    A. Red marks can occur.

    B. Residents can only be turned in every two hours.

    C. Wait for the doctor to prescribe a skin lotion.

    D. Report to the charge nurse.

11. A resident has psoriasis. The CNA must take which of the following steps?

    A. Wear a mask before entering the room.

    B. Wear gloves while giving care.

    C. Avoid contact with skin lesions.

    D. Resident treatment must be the same as for other non-infectious residents.

12. A patient looks paler than he usually does. What must a CNA do?

    A. Offer a snack to the patient.

    B. Offer a glass of water.

    C. Asks the patient how he feels and measures his vitals promptly.

    D. Note it and record it.

13. Mrs. V. has a diagnosis (dx) of congestive heart failure (CHF). Which of the following must be in her care plan?

A. Daily AM weight check.
B. Encourage oral fluids.
C. Apply a TED hose after ambulation.
D. Daily exercise for one hour.

14. Mrs. F is admitted to a care facility after hip replacement surgery. Which of the following accurately describes her condition?

A. Chronic.
B. Acute.
C. Pelvic.
D. Obstetric.

15. A CNA finds blood in a patient's IV tube. What must she do?

A. Report to the charge nurse.
B. Change the IV line.
C. Do nothing.
D. Stop the IV.

16. Who recommends a warm or cold application?

A. A CNA
B. A charge nurse
C. A doctor
D. Director of the facility

17. What is the normal urine color?

A. Colorless
B. Amber
C. Red
D. Yellow

18.   What is the appropriate way to record the rectal temperature of a patient?

    A. Hold the thermometer until it's time to remove it.
    B. Take a break.
    C. Attend to other patients and return in two minutes.
    D. Remain in the room until the time to take the temperature.

19.   How must you manage the drainage bags from urinary catheters?

    A. Kept below bladder level.
    B. Change them in every shift.
    C. Fasten them to the bed frame.
    D. Measure the output daily.

20.   Which step you take before recording a patient's vitals?

    A. Greet the patient and introduce yourself.
    B. Gather all relevant equipment.
    C. Wash hands.
    D. All of the above.

21.   A patient is strictly on I/O status. What is vital to measure for this patient?

    A. The patient must not have oral fluids or food.
    B. Measure all liquids the patient has and all urine outputs.
    C. Measure the patient's void before other things in the morning and at night.
    D. Measure all solids and liquids the patient consumes.

22.   What is the purpose of using a pulse oximeter on a patient?

    A. Measure the oxygen saturation of the blood.
    B. Measure the carbon dioxide content of the lungs.
    C. Measure the oxygen content in the heart.
    D. Measure the carbon dioxide levels in the blood.

23. For a 12-hour shift, how frequently do you reposition immobile patients?

    A. Q2 hr.
    B. Q1 hr.
    C. Q4 hr.
    D. Q6 hr.

24. A patient with pneumonia is weak. Which of the following procedures can you expect in his care plan?

    A. Daily liquid intake 700 cc.
    B. ROM exercises several times daily.
    C. Ensuring coughing and deep breathing exercises several times daily.
    D. Ensuring reduced movement to ease chest pain.

25. Which type of precaution is suitable for a patient with C. Diff?

    A. Droplet
    B. Rectal
    C. Standard
    D. Respiratory

26. While charting I/O for a patient, how would you write the total fluid consumption if the patient has taken 6 oz of milk, 9 oz of juice, and 3 oz of coffee for breakfast?

    A. 18 oz of fluids.
    B. 18 fluid oz of liquid.
    C. 540 ml
    D. 450 ml

27. Which of the following are normal aging symptoms?

    A. Incontinence
    B. Memory loss
    C. Slowing of response time
    D. Losing balance

28.   A patient's care plan states the advice from speech therapy to perform a chin tuck while drinking liquids. Why is this necessary?

A. To prevent aspiration.
B. To help breathe.
C. To help swallow.
D. To prevent the patient from drinking thicker liquids.

29.   A patient with a Foley catheter bag wants to walk around the hall. What should you do first?

A. Cover the Foley bag with a clean cloth for privacy.
B. Ensure carrying the bag below the bladder level.
C. Disconnect the tube from the bag.
D. Hook up the bag onto the patient's waist.

30.   What is the best place to measure the carotid pulse?

A. Side of the neck
B. Front of the neck
C. At the wrist
D. At the elbow

31.   A patient evaluates his pain as 10/10, although he appears cheerful. Why should you report the scoring to the charge nurse?

A. It may upset the patient otherwise.
B. Pain is a subjective perception.
C. To indent medications in case the patient needs them.
D. The patient has a drug use history and needs pain meds.

32.   A patient's vitals show 100 HR, 24 RR, and 102.2 fever. What does the patient have?

A. A case of stomach upset from something she ate.
B. Allergy to some medication.
C. A migraine.

D. An Infection.

33.   A resident with a paralyzed right arm can feed himself with which of the following?

    A. Using a bib.
    B. Sling support.
    C. With the help of an arm brace.
    D. Using a plate guard.

34.   To prevent pressure ulcers, what is the valid method?

    A. Use a gel or a foam pad on top of the mattress.
    B. Brush the patient's dentures regularly.
    C. Change position every four hours.
    D. Increase the dose of vitamin C.

35.   What component of nursing care includes a button hook and a sock assist?

    A. ADL
    B. Prosthetic mobility
    C. Restorative and rehabilitative care
    D. Disability care

36.   How will you position yourself to assist a client in learning to use a cane?

    A. Stand in front of the client on the weak side.
    B. Stand slightly behind the client on the weak side.
    C. Stand one foot from the weaker side.
    D. Stand one foot from the stronger side.

37.   What is the aim of bladder training?

    A. To prevent UTI from indwelling catheters.
    B. To stop catheter use.
    C. To avoid skin issues due to incontinence.
    D. To obtain voluntary urinary control.

38. A resident is screaming and yelling profanities. What is the first step of action for a nurse aide?

    A. Call the supervisor nurse.
    B. Ask the resident to settle down.
    C. Call the resident's family members.
    D. Restrain the resident to prevent self and patient harm.

39. How does self-care help residents with emotional and mental health?

    A. Providing more physical activity.
    B. Ensuring they can control their routines.
    C. Giving a feeling of independence.
    D. Happy to help reduce your workload.

40. What is a helpful listening approach for communication?

    A. Standing 5 feet away from the resident
    B. Offering advice
    C. Avoiding eye contact
    D. Sitting beside the resident

41. A disoriented patient implores to be allowed to go home. What should be your best response?

    A. Stimulate the patient to discuss their home and family.
    B. Say that the facility is their home.
    C. Assure that you will take them to their house later.
    D. Engage the patient in some activity.

42. What do you portray by empathizing with patients?

    A. Feel pity.
    B. Put yourself in others' place.
    C. Allow them to be in bed.
    D. Help them to lift up their moods.

43. Which of these is valid for all behavior?

    A. It means something for the individual.
    B. It has implications for the psychologist.
    C. It is significant to the observer.
    D. It has meaning for the speaker.

44. A culturally diverse client can have distinct views on which of the following?

    A. Food
    B. Religion
    C. Clothing
    D. All of the above

45. What should be the response to a client who asks the nurse aide if she could have a few minutes to pray before her bath?

    A. Bath is a priority.
    B. Bathe the client anyway.
    C. Tell the client to wait until the clergy visit.
    D. Allow some moments to pray.

46. What should be your response to a patient with deafness who repeatedly turns the call light on?

    A. Complaint to the charge nurse about the attention-seeking behavior of the patient
    B. Show the patient to use the call light less often.
    C. Speak loudly through the intercom.
    D. Listen patiently to what the patient needs.

47. What should be the first step before leaving a newly admitted ambulatory client?

    A. Ask if he is hungry.
    B. Inspect his mouth.
    C. Assess intake output.

D. Ensure he knows how to use the call light.

48.   What is the best way to communicate with a client who only speaks and understands a foreign language?

A. Use nonverbal language.
B. Listen carefully and say nothing.
C. Speak slowly.
D. Ask for an interpreter's help.

49.   How should you address a female client?

A. Ma'am
B. Miss
C. By her surname
D. By her first name

50.   A confused patient ambles into other residents' rooms. What should be the appropriate action?

A. Issue a restraint order.
B. Use a barrier to contain the patient.
C. Ask the nurse for sedation.
D. Spend time with the patient and supervise movements.

51.   What is the appropriate technique if a client wants a copy of his medical records?

A. Make a copy and give it to the client.
B. Tell the family about the client's request.
C. Inform the supervisor and provide the record release form.
D. Clients cannot directly have copies of medical records.

52.   What should you do if a client refuses to eat vegetables?

A. Cajole them to have a little.
B. Inform the charge nurse about dietary concerns.
C. Ask the dietician to increase the vegetable content of their dish.

D. Withhold desserts until they finish the vegetables.

53. What would you do if asked to sign a client's will?

    A. Refuse and inform the family.
    B. Refer to someone to arrange for a witness.
    C. Help the client by arranging for case management.
    D. Agree without taking any compensation.

54. A client gives you a $20 bill as a token for your services. What should be your response?

    A. Refuse the offer politely.
    B. Ask the nurse for an appropriate response.
    C. Accept it, not wanting to upset the client.
    D. Accept it and buy something for the team.

55. An individual who claims to be the client's relative but is not on the client's list of people approved to know the client's condition rings and asks about the client's latest status. What should be your response?

    A. "He is in a coma."
    B. "I must add your name to the list."
    C. "Give me your contact information to have someone get back to you."
    D. "I cannot confirm or deny any such individual."

56. Which action do CNAs not perform while arranging clients' rooms?

    A. Adjust the backrest as ordered.
    B. Check the position of the call bell.
    C. Give medicines.
    D. Adjust the light.

57. Which is valid concerning hospital stays?

    A. One week
    B. As long as needed

C. A few days

D. Three days

58.   Which is not a CNA's duty?

A. Insert catheters.

B. Ensure adequate drainage of the catheter.

C. Prevent infection.

D. Record urine output.

59.   Which of the following is important to communicate during a job interview?

A. Credentials

B. Remuneration expectation

C. Childcare requirements

D. Scheduling issues

60.   Which of the following a CNA manifests when she shows interest and concern for her patients?

A. Honesty

B. Accuracy

C. Teamwork

D. Caring

This ends your time for the first practice test. Answers to the questions are in Answer Explanations. The next chapter presents you with the practice test 2.

Answer Key

Q.	1	2	3	4	5	6	7	8	9	10
A.	D	A	D	C	A	C	D	B	D	D

Q.	11	12	13	14	15	16	17	18	19	20
A.	D	C	A	B	A	C	D	D	A	D

Q.	21	22	23	24	25	26	27	28	29	30
A.	B	A	A	C	B	C	C	A	B	A

Q.	31	32	33	34	35	36	37	38	39	40
A.	B	D	D	A	C	B	D	A	B	D

Q.	41	42	43	44	45	46	47	48	49	50
A.	A	B	A	D	D	D	D	B	C	D

Q.	51	52	53	54	55	56	57	58	59	60
A.	C	B	B	A	C	C	B	A	A	D

Answer Explanations

1. D. Soft Toothettes soaked in a solution cleanse the mouth and oral cavity. A Toothette removes food particles and thick saliva from a dry mouth. It lowers infection risk.

2. A. Assist the patient to dress from their weakest side as it supports the affected side and helps maintain the patient's balance.

3. D. Apply a little lotion after bathing to moisturize. Excess quantities, particularly in interdigital areas, may induce perspiration, skin maceration, breakdown, and infection.

4. C. We need to drink water in between morsels throughout the meal.

5. A. The question asked is NOT a familiar problem. A care facility gives consistent patient nutrition.

6. C. Adult patients should void 6–hourly.

7. D. Position for receiving an enema is Left Sim's.

8. B. Clean female perineum from front to back to prevent anal contamination of urethra.

9. D. All of the above.

10. D. Red areas can herald skin breakdown due to pressure and poor circulation. Change posture every two hours if immobile, avoid massaging, and prevent dampness and urine or fecal contamination. Observe the area and report to the charge nurse.

11. D. Psoriasis is non-infectious. It is an autoimmune disease like lupus, celiac disease, and type 1 diabetes in which the patient's immune system attacks healthy tissues.

12. C. Measure vitals if the patient's condition changes, and ask how they feel. Observe, document, and report the findings.

13. A. CHF is a chronic overload of the heart. The patients must not be over-exercised or given excessive fluids. Monitor their weights at the same time and record it accurately. A sudden increase may suggest fluid accumulation that can strain the heart and lungs. Note and report.

14. B. An acute condition like diarrhea, flu, broken bones, etc., appears suddenly. A chronic condition persists. Pelvic conditions are related to the pelvis, and obstetrics pertains to pregnancy and childbirth.

15. A. The IV tube must be clear, and the site must be dry and clean. Report blood in the tube.

16. C. A doctor must order all forms of treatment, including hot and cold compresses.

17. D. Normal urine color is pale yellow. Colorless urine can indicate excess fluid intake. Amber-colored urine can indicate dehydration, and red urine can be due to food, kidney, or prostate diseases.

18. D. Taking a rectal temperature is the most accurate means to record temperature. With the patient in Sim's position, gently insert the rectal thermometer 1"–2" into the rectum. Hold it in place for two minutes to prevent it from being ejected or moving into the rectum.

19. A. Drainage bags from Foley catheters must be kept below bladder level to help drain urine and prevent backflow.

20. D. Greet the patient and introduce yourself, wash hands, explain the procedure, and provide privacy.

21. B. I/O refers to measuring all liquid intake and output. Liquid measurements are in cc or ml.

22. A. Pulse oximetry checks blood oxygen saturation noninvasively.

23. A. The minimum time interval for turning an immobile patient is once every two hours.

24. C. Patients with pneumonia must receive respiratory care, such as back massaging, breathing exercises, and coughing out sputum.

25. B. A patient with C. Diff infection has diarrhea. Take rectal precautions like hand hygiene with soap and water, gown, and gloves before giving patient care. Bag used linens. Visitors are not recommended to prevent the spread of infection.

26. C. Fluid can be charted using cc or ml as measuring units. 18 oz of fluid is 540 ml (1 oz = 30 ml).

27. C. Slower response time is an age-related occurrence due to the degeneration of nerve cells without being regenerateD. Others are not part of normal aging.

28. A. Speech therapy commonly recommends aspiration prevention methods. Chin tuck prevents aspiration and helps the food to pass into the esophagus and not the trachea while swallowing.

29. B. Avoid disconnecting a Foley catheter unless ordered by the doctor. Hooking it higher than the bladder level causes urinary backflow into the bladder, increasing risks for infection. Covering it for cosmetic purposes is unnecessary. A bag under the bladder level is a prerequisite to prevent infection.

30. A. Carotid pulse is felt with two fingers at the side of the neck.

31. B. Pain is subjective, with cultural expressions and individual thresholds.

32. D. Tachycardia (raised HR), tachypnea (raised RR), and fever suggest infection.

33. D. Using a plate guard helps the resident to feed himself.

34. A. Place a gel or a foam pad on top of the mattress.

35. C. A part of the restorative care.

36. B. Stand slightly behind the client on the weak side.

37. D. Aim to restore voluntary bladder control.

38. A. The nurse can guide and direct the action, including giving medications to calm the patient.

39. B. A sense of independence and an improved outlook boost emotional health.

40. D. Patients feel reassured and connected when staff members sit near them, face the patient, and have eye contact while interacting whenever feasible.

41. A. Patients with dementia can occasionally recall memories. Validate them by asking the patient to recall as much as they remember. Often, this is all the patient wants.

42. B. Empathy is the ability to understand what the other person is feeling or experiencing.

43. A. Behaviors must be interpreted from the client's perspective. Patients with dementia are aware of things uncomfortable to them. Family members can help understand behavioral nuances.

44. D. A culturally diverse client can have unique viewpoints on all of these factors.

45. D. Give the patient some private moment to pray. It is an ethically proper action, and an individual's religious and cultural beliefs are legally protected.

46. D. Listen patiently to patient needs.

47. D. Ensure he knows how to use the call light before leaving him alone.

48. B. Listen carefully and say nothing.

49. C. Address a female client by her surname.

50. D. Residents have the right to freedom from physical and chemical restraints.

51. C. Resident's rights to full disclosure of health information and treatment entail they can consent to release information unless incapacitated.

52. B. The right to have freedom of choice and participation in care planning by patients means CNAs can encourage them to eat nutritionally balanced meals but not force them.

53. B. While residents have the right to manage their funds, CNAs cannot engage in patient's legal matters.

54. A. Accepting gifts or cash affects the client-nurse boundary and may call for disciplinary action against a CNA.

55. C. According to HIPPA, patients can restrict who can have access to their health information. Care facilities can confirm patient admission but not medical information.

56. C. CNAs cannot administer medicines.

57. B. Patients' in-hospital stay depends on their condition.

58. A. Interventions are not in the CNA job description.

59. A. Showing appropriate qualifications is essential to job interviews.

60. D. Nursing is all about patient caring.

Chapter Seven: Practice Test 2

The full-length practice test consists of 60 questions with 90 minutes to complete.

1.   What is the next step for a patient on a bowel regimen who had no motions for the last four days?

    A. Report to the nurse.
    B. Give the patient fruit juice with Miralax.
    C. This is normal.
    D. Encourage drinking more water.

2.   What area of a female patient could get contaminated if a CNA does not perform perineal care from front to back?

    A. Rectum
    B. Cervix
    C. Urinary meatus
    D. Uvula

3.   What should be your action if a diabetic patient finishes only 20% of his meal?

    A. Nothing; the patient is probably not hungry.
    B. Report to the nurse.
    C. Chart it for the nurse to see.
    D. Try again with dinner.

4. A patient on a clear liquid diet for an upcoming colonoscopy is expected to have which of the following on his tray?

    A. Water, coffee, and milk
    B. Soup, coffee, and tea
    C. Jello, Sprite, and water
    D. Milk, tea, and soda

5. A client with Alzheimer's refuses dinner. What should be appropriate to tell her?

    A. "The doctor will be worried if you refuse food."
    B. "I respect your decision." Inform the charge nurse thereafter.
    C. "It is unhealthy not to eat."
    D. "Please eat for your family's sake."

6. While transferring a patient with a gait belt, he starts to fall. What should you do?

    A. Catch the patient by the gait belt, leaning forward.
    B. Allow the patient to slip and then lift him up.
    C. Shout for assistance.
    D. Grab the belt to lower the patient slowly to the ground, resting most of the weight on your legs.

7. What type of diet is suitable for a patient with dysphagia?

    A. Pureed
    B. Clear liquid
    C. Regular
    D. Mechanical soft

8. A resident who eats slowly regularly leaves her post-lunch PT sessions, which last for an hour, incomplete. What should you do?

    A. Take the patient to her lunch earlier to allow her to get full PT sessions.
    B. Tell the patient that you will assist her to eat faster.
    C. Report the physical therapist to the supervisor.

D. The patient can eat for as long as she wants.

9.   What should you do if family members of an Alzheimer's patient remain in the room for most of your shift, preventing you from bathing the patient?

   A. Tell the charge nurse.
   B. Ask the patient to call you once the visitors leave.
   C. Schedule the bath first thing the following day.
   D. Ask the visitors to step outside until the bath is complete.

10.   When should a patient eat breakfast after receiving the morning dose of short-acting insulin?

   A. 30 minutes
   B. One hour
   C. ASAP
   D. 15 minutes

11.   What should you chart after giving 8 oz of water to a patient?

   A. 8 oz of water
   B. 80 cc of water
   C. 80 ml of water
   D. 240 ml of water

12.   What should you immediately assess in a diabetes patient with disorientation and sweating?

   A. Blood pressure
   B. Respiratory rate
   C. Heart rate
   D. Blood sugar

13.   Which of the following needs contact precaution?

   A. Pneumonia

B. MRSA
C. Covid 19
D. TB

14. Which of the following is subjective information?

A. Temperature 101.5°F
B. Eggs for breakfast
C. BP 120/90
D. Pain level 7/10

15. In which condition can you expect dark stools?

A. Hepatitis
B. Appendicitis
C. GI bleed
D. Gastroenteritis

16. What is the rate of CPR on an adult patient?

A. 100–120 compressions/minute
B. 75–100 compressions/minute
C. 85–140 compressions/minute
D. 150–200 compressions/minute

17. Which arm is proper to record BP in a patient with a left-sided mastectomy?

A. Only the right arm.
B. Only the left arm.
C. Any arm.
D. Only on the lower limbs.

18. What is the proper place to tie a restraint for a patient having a restraint order?

A. The lower bed rail.

B. The upper bed rail.
C. The head of bed.
D. The bedframe.

19.   Why is it important to avoid wrinkles in bedsheets?

A. They may entangle the patient's feet.
B. Wrinkles are not neat.
C. To prevent bedsores.
D. To prevent falls.

20.   What is the best way to ensure patient safety while meeting them on your shift?

A. Check their charts.
B. Have them tell you their names.
C. Check whether the patient's name and the room number are on the patient's door.
D. Ask them to tell you their names and DOBs and verify them against those on their armband.

21.   What is the best practice to turn a patient with a Foley catheter?

A. Hang the catheter to the bedframe.
B. Ask the patient to hold the catheter while you turn them.
C. Tape the catheter to the inner thigh.
D. Tape the catheter to the outer thigh.

22.   Which of the following occurs in a patient with a stroke?

A. Foaming at the mouth
B. Involuntary urination
C. Unilateral drooping of the face
D. Rolling back of eyes

23. Which is the best approach to prevent the spread of germs?

     A. Wearing a mask and gloves for patient care
     B. Handwashing before and after patient care
     C. Wearing gloves for patient care
     D. Wearing a gown, mask, and gloves for patient care

24. A patient using underwear suffers from incontinence. Which method is appropriate for him?

     A. Assisting him to visit the toilet frequently
     B. Giving him less fluids
     C. Medications to void the bladder fully
     D. Using a Foley catheter

25. What is the purpose of a fracture-type bedpan?

     A. To raise the buttocks.
     B. To maintain spinal alignment.
     C. Women patients.
     D. Both a and b.

26. How many fingers can you insert under a wrist restraint?

     A. 3
     B. 4
     C. 2
     D. 0

27. What is the proper method to count respirations?

     A. Read chest rises for 10 seconds and multiply it by 6.
     B. Read chest rises for 60 seconds.
     C. Count to 60 using a stethoscope on the chest.
     D. Read chest rises for 30 seconds and multiply it by 2.

28. What should you use to transfer a patient with generalized weakness from the bed to a chair?

    A. Sliding board
    B. Sit-to-stand lift
    C. Hoyer lift
    D. Gait belt

29. A resident aged 75 years is otherwise pleasant. You find her agitated, thrashing and knocking, and failing to recognize the staff. What is the likely cause of her cognitive delays?

    A. Hunger
    B. Headache
    C. UTI
    D. Sinus infection

30. Which of these is essential for diabetic care?

    A. Keep the feet dry and warm with dry, clean socks.
    B. Clip the nails short for hygiene.
    C. Daily soaking for dry, calloused feet.
    D. Provide a heating pad for cold extremities.

31. Which of these is true for side rails?

    A. Raise all four side rails for patient safety.
    B. Raise the side rails when the patient is sleeping.
    C. Raise side rails on one side at a time.
    D. Raise side rails on both sides.

32. What is the risk for a bedbound patient?

    A. Neck paralysis
    B. Atrophy
    C. Polydipsia
    D. Dysphasia

33. How do you keep hearing aids when not in use?

    A. Left turned on
    B. In the patient's pocket
    C. Kept without the battery
    D. On the bedside table

34. How would you manage a patient walking back and forth in a hall?

    A. Walk with him.
    B. Restrain him.
    C. Observe him.
    D. Report him.

35. How best to use a cane with weakness on one side of the body?

    A. Both sides, depending on the client's feelings.
    B. Strong side.
    C. Weaker side.
    D. Alternately, on the stronger and weaker sides.

36. What is the linen spread from the client's shoulder to the thighs?

    A. Underpad
    B. Drawsheet
    C. Spread
    D. A sheet

37. Which is a special device to control contractures?

    A. Handroll
    B. Air mattress
    C. Doppler
    D. Manometer

38.   What is the best response to an anxious patient in a new setting?

A. Speak calmly and show composed and comforting behavior.
B. Allow the patient to re-focus and reorganize in private.
C. Distract by turning the radio or TV on.
D. Light up the room to give a cheery feel.

39.   How do you respond to a client who wants to talk about impending death?

A. Allow him to express his feelings if he is willing to.
B. Talk about how you overcame your personal grief.
C. Distract the patient.
D. Tell him that we all will die someday.

40.   Which is not a cause for constipation?

A. Depression
B. High-fat meals
C. Anxiety
D. Increased intestinal motility

41.   Which is not a proper way to deal with caregiving stress?

A. Engage in a hobby.
B. Learn something new.
C. Talk to your coworker about clients to vent your feelings.
D. Outdoor exercises.

42.   A family member is angry because her close one is sad. What should be your best response?

A. Listen carefully and ensure that you will talk to the nurse.
B. Ask her to submit her complaints in writing.
C. Tell her that you will allow her privacy to help her calm down.
D. State that you cannot discuss the resident's care.

43. What is appropriate care for a patient with Alzheimer's who seems sad and silent?

    A. Talk to him.
    B. Observe him for non-verbal cues.
    C. Change subjects until he starts talking.
    D. Tell him not to worry.

44. Which is not part of Hospice care?

    A. Dying is part of a life cycle.
    B. The family should not witness the dying process.
    C. Care for the dying person involves physical, emotional, and spiritual needs.
    D. Care for the dying person seeks to alleviate pain.

45. Which of these has no impact on an individual's feelings about death?

    A. Culture
    B. Religion
    C. Financial condition
    D. Present quality of life

46. How would you best interact with a young, permanently disabled resident who seems indifferent to her condition?

    A. Address her by her name.
    B. Include her in her care plan.
    C. Serve her meals first.
    D. Doing her care for her.

47. Why is effective communication a crucial aspect of a nurse aide's job?

    A. Nurse aides are front-line caregivers in most healthcare settings.
    B. Nurse aides should communicate patient information to others in the facility.
    C. The nurse aide's role is task completion and not communication.
    D. Nurse aides should not mediate between doctor-patient communication.

48. Which of the following is an example of body language?

    A. Suggesting advice and perspectives
    B. Using gestures and facial expressions
    C. Writing down the message
    D. Sharing of feelings and concerns

49. Which type of nonverbal communication is best demonstrated when a nurse aide beams and shakes her head while sitting with a client?

    A. Encourages the client to talk
    B. Shows discomfort to listen to the client
    C. Agrees with the client totally
    D. She has no work to do

50. Who is it appropriate to share a patient's personal information with?

    A. The spouse.
    B. The roommate.
    C. The patient's children.
    D. The nursing assistant on the next shift.

51. Which of these describes restorative nursing?

    A. Not a CNA's obligation.
    B. The patient can be discharged and do self-care.
    C. Patients gain and maintain their functionality.
    D. CNA hands over patient care duties to family members.

52. Which of these depict the right to telephone privileges?

    A. Each patient has rights to phone access and privacy.
    B. Patients can use telephones at the facility, but they must have their own.
    C. Telephone use requires the caregiver's supervision.
    D. The use of telephones is allowed during scheduled times.

53.	Which of these does not show caring behavior?

   A. Asking a co-worker to share your duty so that you do not miss lunch
   B. Listening to an anxious patient
   C. Staying up with a lonely patient
   D. Comforting a patient who is crying

54.	What is the appropriate action for a 78-year-old patient with multiple bruises at various healing stages on his body?

   A. Report possible abuse on an abuse hotline.
   B. Report possible abuse to the police.
   C. The bruises can be due to the skin fragility of old age.
   D. It could be due to medications like blood thinners.

55.	A patient's daughter requests you not to divulge information about cancer relapse to the patient. How should you respond?

   A. Listen to the daughter.
   B. Embolden her to tell the patient who has a right to know.
   C. Tell her to inform the patient right away, or you will report abuse.
   D. Tell her that she is wrong to withhold information, but you will listen to her.

56.	What should you do if you're unable to work due to illness?

   A. Wait until the charge nurse phones you.
   B. Call the charge nurse an hour before the shift starts.
   C. Contact the supervisor promptly.
   D. Arrange for someone to cover your shift.

57.	What work procedure is followed if you and your co-worker are assigned bathing and vital signs recording, respectively?

   A. Team
   B. Patient-centered
   C. Modular
   D. Primary

58.   Which of these is the CNA's responsibility?

   A. Plan client care.
   B. Perform tasks assigned by the charge nurse.
   C. Never ask for help during work.
   D. Comparing assignments with colleagues.

59.   Which of these is a reason for a CNA to refuse work?

   A. The client is difficult.
   B. Another individual can do the task.
   C. She has not been trained to do the work.
   D. Her shift is ending.

60.   Who is supervised by an RN?

   A. Doctors
   B. Residents
   C. Administration
   D. Nursing assistants

It is time to stop taking practice test 2. Before moving to practice test 3, evaluate your test performance by referring to answers to these questions in Answer Explanations.

Answer Key

Q.	1	2	3	4	5	6	7	8	9	10
A.	A	C	B	C	B	A	D	A	D	B

Q.	11	12	13	14	15	16	17	18	19	20
A.	D	C	A	D	C	A	A	D	C	D

Q.	21	22	23	24	25	26	27	28	29	30
A.	C	C	B	A	D	C	B	D	C	A

Q.	31	32	33	34	35	36	37	38	39	40
A.	D	B	C	C	B	B	A	A	A	D

Q.	41	42	43	44	45	46	47	48	49	50
A.	C	A	B	B	C	B	A	B	A	D

Q.	51	52	53	54	55	56	57	58	59	60
A.	C	A	A	A	B	C	C	B	C	D

Answer Explanations

1. A. A bowel regimen enhances bowel movements. Report lack of bowel movements for four days to the nurse.

2. C. Back-to-front strokes can spread fecal bacteria from the rectum to the urinary meatus.

3. B. Promptly report to the nurse to avert hypoglycemia.

4. C. Patients should have clear transparent fluids at room temperature (72°F–78°F) before colonoscopy. Soup and milk are opaque. Jello is liquid at room temperature.

5. B. Alzheimer's patients may refuse or forget to eat; note the cause for not eating and report the nurse.

6. A. Avoid leaning forward. Use proper body mechanics to Grab the belt and lower the patient slowly to the ground, putting most of the weight on your legs.

7. D. Dysphagia is difficulty in swallowing. Mechanical soft food and thickened liquids (to prevent choking on thin liquids) facilitate swallowing.

8. A. ADLs facilitate self-care routines for the residents. While option b offsets the concept, set an earlier time to finish the meal.

9. D. Take charge of a patient's privacy and accomplish your tasks within an acceptable time.

10. B. MRSA is a skin infection spreading through skin contact. Others are respiratory infections.

11. D. We can feel pain, which is subjective.

12. C. Dark tarry stools frequently indicate GI tract bleeding; report to the nurse.

13. A. According to the American Heart Association, the proper CPR rate is 100–120 compressions/minute to perfuse the brain and other tissue during cardiac arrest.

14. D. We can feel pain, which is subjective.

15. C. Dark tarry stools frequently indicate GI tract bleeding; report to the nurse.

16. A. According to the American Heart Association, the proper CPR rate is 100–120 compressions/minute to perfuse the brain and other tissue during cardiac arrest.

17. A. Measuring the BP on the affected side increases the risk for cellulitis and lymphedema in post-surgery breast cancer.

18. D. The bed rails are movable; the restraints can become loose or too tight, endangering the Patient or staff. Bedframes are more suitable.

19. C. Decubitus ulcer can occur following prolonged bed rest. Wrinkles in the sheets can cause skin breakdown, leading to decubitus ulcers.

20. D. The Patient's name on their door is a HIPAA violation. Checking their chart is not infallible. Disoriented patients may confuse their names. Ask patients to tell you their names and DOBs and verify them against those on their armbands.

21. C. Secure the Foley catheter to the upper inner thigh unless contraindicated.

22. C. Stroke can present with asymmetrical face drooping.

23. B. Hand washing is the best hand hygiene in a healthcare setting; do it before and after patient care and when the hands are soiled.

24. A. Assist incontinent patients in using the restroom throughout the day to prevent the bladder from getting too full.

25. D. Fracture pans are used for weaker individuals who cannot lift their hips and those who need strict spinal alignment.

26. C. Sliding two fingers under the wrist restraint ensures they are not too tight or loose. Assess at least after every two hours.

27. B. Observe and count the chest rises for a full 60 seconds while counting respirations to avoid variations in the number of times a patient may actually breathe per minute. Avoid counting RR using a stethoscope.

28. D. Repositioning from one place to another, such as a bed to chair, chair to bed, or bed to wheelchair, requires using a gait belt to assist patients who are weak but not bedbound.

29. C. After age 65, UTI is common and can cause sudden cognitive delays. Report to the charge nurse.

30. A. Inspect the feet daily and keep them clean and dry because diabetic patients with neuropathy may lack foot sensations and have infections and delayed wound healing.

31. D. Raise the top side rails at all times. Raising four side rails can be considered a restraint and is acceptable while transporting a patient on the beD.

32. B. Muscle atrophy is muscle wasting, which happens quickly in immobile patients. ROM and PROM can check atrophy.

33. C. Remove the battery of hearing aids when not in use.

34. C. Watch the client.

35. B. Use the cane on the unaffected side.

36. B. The linen spread from the client's shoulder to the thighs is a draw sheet.

37. A. The handroll is a special device to control contractures.

38. A. Reduced stimuli work best to alleviate anxiety. The other options trigger a tense situation further, aggravating anxiousness.

39. A. Validate the patient's concern by allowing him to talk willingly on a subject he wishes to discuss.

40. D. Increased motility can increase stool frequency.

41. C. Sharing identical problems is therapeutic. Divulging information about residents violates privacy.

42. A. Reassure the individual. Other methods stall communication and leave the issue unsolved.

43. B. Observe his nonverbal cues.

44. B. The dying person must be with family and other support systems.

45. C. All, except financial conditions, can impact beliefs about death.

46. B. Include the client in her care plan to feel in control.

47. A. Nurse aides are front-line caregivers and intermediaries between doctors and patients.

48. B. Nonverbal body language is expressed through gestures and facial expressions.

49. A. The nurse aide gives optimistic company to the client.

50. D. Share relevant information with the next shift's CNA to help patient care. According to HIPAA, patients can decide who will receive their medical information.

51. C. Patients gain and maintain their functionality and well-being with restorative care.

52. A. Patients have the right to telephone access and privacy to use it.

53. A. CNAs must finish scheduled tasks on the care plan. Time may not know its boundaries in a healthcare profession.

54. A. Skin bruises occur due to aging, but various stages of healing express chronic abuse. Report any possible abuse.

55. B. Withholding patient information from them is wrong and unethical.

56. C. Contact the supervisor promptly.

57. C. Modular nursing emerged from team nursing to simplify inpatient and outpatient care. RNs lead geographic modules of a patient care unit. Module caretakers are always the same, with available medication, supplies, and linens. The team comprises RNs, LPNs, and nursing assistants.

58. B. CNAs do assigned tasks by the charge nurse.

59. C. Do tasks included in your training.

60. D. RNs supervise the nursing assistants who provide basic care and help patients with ADLs.

Chapter Eight: Practice Test 3

The test has 60 questions with 90 minutes.

1.   Which of the following essential bathing needs is neglected by caregivers and facilities?

  A. Cultural variations of bathing frequency.
  B. Rinsing and drying must be thorough.
  C. The caregiver must use proper body mechanics to avoid injury.
  D. Safe bath water temperature.

2.   Which of these is the facility's decision for providing nail care?

  A. Nail care is best provided sitting, although residents can also be in bed.
  B. Report any alteration of nail beds to the nurse.
  C. The policy of cutting toenails can vary.
  D. Soak the nails for 10 minutes before starting.

3.   Which of these is not valid for denture care?

  A. Keep them in cold water.
  B. They are expensive and fragile.
  C. They slip when wet.
  D. Residents are responsible for their dentures.

4. Which of these are unsafe procedures for nonambulatory patients?

   A. Routine check-up for pressure sores.
   B. Two-hourly repositioning.
   C. Keeping the residents clean and dry.
   D. Re-positioning once per shift.

5. What is Hoyer Lift's purpose?

   A. Transferring patients from bed to chair.
   B. Transferring patients from bed to stretcher.
   C. Moving patients into the car.
   D. Moving patients into the bathtub.

6. Which of these is ensured for bathing besides safety and privacy?

   A. Quietness
   B. Security
   C. Dimmed setting
   D. Swiftness

7. Tooth decay, foul odor, and cracks in the mouth signify which condition?

   A. Dehydration
   B. Insufficient toothpaste use
   C. Wet mouth
   D. Dry mouth

8. Which essential hair care necessity is overlooked?

   A. Age
   B. Weather
   C. Ethnicity
   D. Duration of stay

9. Which condition denotes small, watery leakage of stools?

   A. Fecal impaction
   B. Diarrhea
   C. Medicine side effect
   D. Weak muscle tone

10. What does "O2 per N/C @3L, orthopnea posture as needed" suggest for you in a care plan?

    A. Three–hourly oral care
    B. Client orientation at @3 to the orthopedic unit
    C. Maintain Fowler's position for the patient
    D. Three-hourly ambulation

11. What is caused by smoking?

    A. Pneumonia
    B. Heart attack
    C. Vitamin C deficiency
    D. All of the above

12. What is the appropriate action if a patient on oxygen via nasal cannula (NC) has an O2 saturation of 85%?

    A. Increase O2 flow.
    B. Report to the nurse.
    C. Replace NC with a mask.
    D. Ask the patient to breathe more frequently.

13. What is a colostomy opening on the skin called?

    A. Stoma
    B. Orifice
    C. Rectum
    D. Cloaca

14. Which of these is valid for the circulatory system anatomy?

    A. Blood and lymph vessels, spleen
    B. Blood vessels, heart, lungs
    C. Heart, arteries, veins, capillaries
    D. Heart, pulmonary vessels, lungs

15. Which condition is promptly reported?

    A. BP: 90/40
    B. HR: 90
    C. RR: 15
    D. Temperature: 99.4°

16. Which of these must be changed carefully to avoid accidental pricks by used needles?

    A. Used bed linens
    B. Used washcloths
    C. Patients' clothing
    D. Trash bags

17. What {L}sided hemiplegia means?

    A. L arm contracture
    B. L arm and leg twitchings
    C. L-side body paralysis
    D. L arm rashes

18. What does postpartum mean?

    A. Immediately preceding birth
    B. Immediately after birth
    C. Immediately before death
    D. Immediately after death

19.   What does NPO after midnight signify?

A. Frequent snacking.
B. Remove the water pitcher after midnight.
C. Document all intake and output.
D. Assess pain.

20.   Which situation is inappropriate for alcohol-based hand rub?

A. After handling patients' clothes
B. After ambulating patients
C. Unavailability of soap and water
D. Observable dirt in the hands

21.   What information is necessary for a resident who is pale, sweaty, and confused after a morning dose of insulin?

A. Excessive sugary food consumption
B. Distractions caused by visitors
C. Ate his breakfast
D. He has diabetes

22.   Which part of anatomy evacuates stool after an ileostomy surgery?

A. Colon
B. Ilium
C. Anus
D. Stomach

23.   Which procedure helps in the accurate estimation of resident weight?

A. Compare with another scale
B. At the same time every day
C. After a meal
D. Three hours post-meals

24. What is the first step for measuring vital signs?

   A. Wash your hands.
   B. Greet and introduce yourself.
   C. Find appropriate equipment.
   D. All of the above.

25. Which of these ensures blood circulation?

   A. ROM
   B. Back massage
   C. Repositioning the patient frequently
   D. All of the above

26. What is the best approach if a patient on IV complains of hand pain and has puffy hands?

   A. Report to the floor nurse.
   B. Apply an ice pack.
   C. Massage the hand.
   D. Reassure the patient.

27. The brain belongs to which part of the human system?

   A. Endocrine
   B. Nervous
   C. Locomotor
   D. Exocrine

28. What should be the source of most of our calories?

   A. Carbohydrates
   B. Fats
   C. Proteins
   D. Vitamins

29.   What is ongoing education?

    A. Learning new developments
    B. Maintain professional standard
    C. Required for recertification in many states
    D. All of the above

30.   Which is not true for blindness?

    A. Ask a blind person if he needs assistance before helping him.
    B. Diabetes can cause blindness.
    C. Identify yourself before touching a blind individual.
    D. Most blind people are visionless.

31.   What is the professional dress code?

    A. Jewelry reflects a cheerful personality.
    B. Carefully manicured nails.
    C. Sandals, T-shirts, and name tags.
    D. Clean, wrinkle-free uniforms, clipped fingernails.

32.   What should you notice before serving the meal trays?

    A. Check armbands routinely.
    B. Check food temperature.
    C. Ask about diet restrictions.
    D. Inquire whether the patient is hungry.

33.   Which condition is helped by frequently turning the client?

    A. Clubbing
    B. Nausea
    C. Heart disease
    D. Pressure injuries

34. Which is most critical to prevent skin breakdown?

    A. Air-dry the skin
    B. Moisturize the skin
    C. Ambulate the client once daily
    D. Reposition the client 2-hourly

35. What is the best way to promote independence when bathing a client after a stroke?

    A. Give a complete bath only when he wants.
    B. Motivate him for self-care and assist as needed.
    C. Leave him alone.
    D. Wash his hands only.

36. How can you help prevent pressure injuries?

    A. Repositioning every 4 hours
    B. Massaging reddened areas on the skin
    C. Keeping linens dry and wrinkle-free
    D. Using soap

37. How would you encourage the independence of a client with arthritis in eating?

    A. Cut the food and feed him.
    B. Insist that he eats without help.
    C. Assist him in cutting the food and using special eating utensils.
    D. Serve pureed food.

38. What is the best response for a resident whose spouse has recently died?

    A. Assemble other residents to divert attention.
    B. Use humor to lighten moods.
    C. Spend time listening to the resident.
    D. Ignore and switch the topic if the resident gets emotional.

39.   What could be the reason for a resident's animosity toward family members?

A. Missing birthdays
B. Missing family meals
C. A feeling of abandonment
D. Spiritual disquiet

40.   How do you respond to a resident's altered mental condition?

A. The resident needs more time and assistance.
B. Prompt reporting to the nurse.
C. Inquire about recent personality changes.
D. Rely on laughter to uplift mood.

41.   How would you assist clients spiritually?

A. Inspire clients to talk about their beliefs.
B. They should focus on exercising.
C. Talk about your beliefs.
D. Avoid discussing religion.

42.   What is likely for a disoriented resident?

A. Has developmental delays
B. Space and temporal confusion
C. Likely to become aggressive
D. Is over 70 years of age

43.   Which one is allowed for a patient on suicide alert?

A. A mirror
B. Album of family pictures
C. Glass vessel with flowers
D. A favorite belt

44. What is needed for postmortem care?

    A. Towels
    B. Bedsheets
    C. Bed bath supplies
    D. Nothing

45. When is postmortem care given?

    A. Five hours after death
    B. No fixed time
    C. Before the onset of rigor mortis
    D. None of the above

46. What is best to talk to visually disabled residents?

    A. Touch the resident before talking
    B. Announce yourself
    C. Talk loudly
    D. Turn on all lights

47. Why is active listening important?

    A. Checks misunderstandings
    B. Effortless
    C. Removes the need for questioning
    D. Gives response time

48. When should you suspect pain even when the resident says she is fine?

    A. She jumbles up language.
    B. She has a high pain threshold.
    C. She takes analgesics.
    D. She is grimacing.

49.   How should you respond to a client who states that "God is punishing me" or "Why me?"

A. Listen and inquire to learn
B. Disagree with her
C. Introduce humor
D. Talk about similar feelings

50.   How do you show respect to a resident?

A. Listening to them
B. Correcting them
C. Agreeing with them
D. Cleaning the mess

51.   Which right would you protect by not discussing residents' condition with a neighbor?

A. Respect
B. Privacy
C. Informed consent
D. Confidentiality

52.   When you bathe a patient who refused the service, you violate which right?

A. Right to refuse treatment
B. Right to privacy
C. Right to complain
D. Right to schedule

53.   What will you do before entering a client's room?

A. Turn the lights on.
B. Identify yourself.
C. Knock on the door.
D. Call the client's name.

54. What is the best action for a patient who suddenly tries to hit you?

    A. Leave the spot and call security.
    B. Retreat and talk calmly.
    C. Hit back the patient.
    D. Ask the nurse about issuing restraint orders.

55. How do you respond to a patient saying, "I overheard the nurse tell my roommate that he has cancer; cancer where? Will he survive?

    A. "It is confidential, but you can talk to him about it."
    B. "He has lung cancer, poor thing."
    C. "Please ask the nurse."
    D. "Why not ask his son tomorrow?"

56. What is appropriate for a patient whose BP record is 200/100? He has no distress.

    A. Notify the nurse.
    B. Measure RR and HR, completing the vitals.
    C. Document the findings.
    D. Ensure the correct size of the BP cuff and recheck.

57. Which of these is a part of a CNA's care plan?

    A. Wound dressing
    B. Notice mental state changes
    C. Bathing assistance
    D. Give IV medicines

58. When are universal precautions practiced?

    A. With fever
    B. With cough
    C. With wounds
    D. For all clients

59.   What are you expected to wear for C. Diff infection?

A. Gown
B. Face shield
C. Surgical mask
D. N95 respirator

60.   What should you do if the client's family desires that you stroll them without a mobile walker? The care plan mentions the client should walk using the rolling walker.

A. Inform the family that the care plan advises using the walker and report to the nurse.
B. Listen to the family.
C. Use a wheelchair for ambulation.
D. The family should ambulate the client without the rolling walker.

It is time to stop taking practice test 3. Before moving to practice test 4, evaluate your test performance by referring to answers to these questions in Answer Explanations.

Answer Key

Q.	1	2	3	4	5	6	7	8	9	10
A.	A	C	D	D	A	B	D	C	A	B

Q.	11	12	13	14	15	16	17	18	19	20
A.	D	B	A	C	A	A	C	B	B	D

Q.	21	22	23	24	25	26	27	28	29	30
A.	A	B	B	D	D	A	B	A	D	D

Q.	31	32	33	34	35	36	37	38	39	40
A.	D	A	D	D	B	C	C	D	C	B

Q.	41	42	43	44	45	46	47	48	49	50
A.	A	B	B	C	C	C	A	D	A	A

Q.	51	52	53	54	55	56	57	58	59	60
A.	D	A	C	B	A	D	C	D	A	A

Answer Explanations

1. A. Consideration of residents' cultural concepts of bathing frequency is a must.

2. C. Many facilities reserve nail care for nurses and doctors; others are CNA's duties.

3. D. Residents cannot care for their dentures.

4. D. Turn patients as frequently as possible, at least every two hours.

5. A. Hoyer Lift, a safety device, is primarily used to transfer patients from bed to chair and back.

6. B. Undressing causes anxiousness and vulnerability. Safety, privacy, and security are prime considerations for ADLs.

7. D. Insufficient saliva encourages the growth of oral bacteria, producing bad breath and tooth rot.

8. C. Racial and cultural considerations are essential for scheduling hair care.

9. A. Small amounts of wet feces on clothes or after defecation suggest fecal impaction. Report to the nurse immediately for possible interventions.

10. B. The patient is on 3L of oxygen through the nasal cannula and may need Fowler posture for short breaths (orthopnea).

11. D. Smoking causes heart attack, stroke, emphysema, COPD, lung cancers, and Vitamin B and C deficiencies.

12. B. CNAs should observe and report and not regulate oxygen flow, which for COPD is regulated at 88%– 92% saturation.

13. A. Cloaca isn't human anatomy; the rectum is the last segment of the large gut, and the orifice is any exterior opening. A stoma is a colostomy opening to the outer surface.

14. C. The circulatory system comprises the heart, arteries, veins, and capillaries.

15. A. BP < 90/60 is hypotension; report sudden drops promptly.

16. A. Carefully change bed linens because procedures with sharps and needles could be performed at the bedside.

17. C. {L} or Left-sided hemiplegia is paralysis of the left side of the body, partial or total.

18. B. Partum means giving birth. The prefix post- means after. Postpartum is the time after delivery.

19. B. NPO means nothing per mouth, including water.

20. D. Observable dirt always requires washing with soap and water.

21. A. Insulin, given to diabetics, can drop blood sugar, causing hypoglycemia, and is connected to meal timings. Late meals can cause hypoglycemia symptoms like sweating, palpitations, and tremors.

22. B. An ileostomy is an opening of the ilium on the lower right side of the body.

23. B. Weigh residents at the same time daily, preferably on the same scale, for accuracy under similar conditions.

24. D. Before measuring vital signs, ensure patient comfort, hand hygiene, and availability of proper equipment.

25. D. Good blood circulation prevents skin breakdown. CNAs can ensure this by performing ROM and PROM, back massage, and turning patients frequently.

26. A. Report to the nurse if patients complain of pain in the IV line or their hands swell up.

27. B. The brain belongs to the nervous system.

28. A. Carbohydrates account for 45%–65% of calories daily.

29. D. Continuing education helps maintain professional standards, obtain re-certification, and know new developments.

30. D. Most blind people have some visual perceptions.

31. D. Each facility has a dress code.

32. A. Always check the clients' ID band of the name tag and match it to the correct food tray to avoid risks like food allergy or fluid restrictions.

33. D. Pressure injuries are prevented by frequent repositioning.

34. D. Reposition the client after every two hours.

35. B. Motivate him for self-care and assist as needed.

36. C. Prevent pressure sores by ensuring linens are dry and wrinkle-free.

37. C. Assist him in cutting the food and using special eating utensils.

38. D. Someone who has lost a loved one may need to express their thoughts and memories. Sitting and holding the resident's hand often soothes them.

39. C. Placing one's care in others' hands and severance from regular life is daunting and not often a choice.

40. B. Subtle mood changes can herald significant mental distress that the resident may not be aware of.

41. A. Patients approach medical treatment with a holistic approach that incorporates spirituality. Discussing spiritual needs and beliefs during illness and adversity may be therapeutic for many.

42. B. Check whether a confused consumer recognizes you in a relaxed and calm manner. Suggesting food items like chicken for dinner can help with spatial

and temporal orientation. Room surroundings with familiar items and pictures may also help.

43. B. Belts, glass, shoelaces, razors, and bedsheets are potential suicide accessories.

44. C. Postmortem care requires washing or cleansing of the deceased with dignity.

45. C. Rigor mortis stiffens the body, complicating postmortem care.

46. C. Speak naturally, addressing the client directly. Never assume patients know your voice. Identify yourself before entering the client's room. Reduce distractions. Tell them when you leave the room.

47. A. Active listening eliminates misunderstandings.

48. D. Grimacing, frowning, and tightened lips are nonverbal pain communication.

49. A. Use active listening to give attention and discernment to the client instead of disagreeing or ignoring her concerns.

50. A. Use active listening to show respect and appreciation.

51. D. HIPAA prohibits divulging patient information with individuals not directly linked to patient care.

52. A. Patients can refuse treatment and complain against the CNA.

53. C. Seek your permission to enter a client's room.

54. B. Don't allow patients to harm you. Step back and reassure. Listen to their emotions and words to understand their actions.

55. A. Maintaining patient confidentiality is crucial.

56. D. Measure BP with the correct cuff size, recheck, and report if BP is still high.

57. C. Bathing assistance is the CNAs' role.

58. D. Universal precautions are for the safety of all clients and staff.

59. A. C. Diff is a GI infection; use gowns for safety.

60. A. Care plans help staff understand client safety requirements. The CNA should follow the care plan and notify the nurse of changes.

Chapter Nine: Practice Test 4

Practice test 4 has 60 questions, which you must answer in 90 minutes.

1.   What should you do if the patient is incontinent just before dinner?

   A. Clean them before taking them to dinner.
   B. Insist they should dine in their room.
   C. Change, take them to eat, and then clean.
   D. Take them to dinner and clean afterward.

2.   What is an essential procedure before bathing?

   A. Soaking the feet
   B. Checking water temperature
   C. Shampooing the hair
   D. Moisturizing the skin

3.   Why is the perineum cleaned after elimination with soap and water?

   A. Removes feces and urine
   B. Prevents soiling of linens
   C. Keeps the area germ-free
   D. Reduces facility's linen-related costs

4.   During PM care of a patient, where should you keep his denture set?

A. Under the pillow
B. Bedside table
C. Sink
D. Denture cup

5.   Which ensures complete privacy?

A. Drawing curtains all around while caregiving
B. Dragging the curtains when there is a roommate
C. Pulling the curtains per the resident's wish
D. Caring with open doors

6.   Which is incorrect for oral care?

A. Proper oral care fights germs
B. Cleans plaque
C. Unsuitable for unconscious patients
D. Required daily

7.   Which is valid for a sitz bath?

A. Given for an hour
B. Immerse the pelvic region in 80°F water
C. The water level is up to the heart
D. It cleans the perineum and relieves pain

8.   Which is the last region cleaned during a bed bath?

A. Armpits
B. Feet
C. Perineum
D. Eyes

9.   What is the next step for a patient refusing a bath?

    A. Report to nurse
    B. Give the bath anyway
    C. Change the care plan
    D. Inform the family

10.   Which is correct for a patient complaining of pain on seeing you?

    A. Take the client outdoors.
    B. Turn the television on.
    C. Soothe the client.
    D. Report to the nurse.

11.   What is the proper step to don a gown to attend isolation patients?

    A. Leave it untied for quicker operations.
    B. Take off the gown before leaving the room.
    C. Doff the gown in the designated dirty area.
    D. Wear it for caring for other patients, reducing laundry costs.

12.   What is the correct way to make an occupied bed?

    A. Raise the rail on the unguarded side.
    B. Keep the bed at the lowest level for patient safety.
    C. Lower both rails before replacing the sheet.
    D. Keep used sheets on the floor.

13.   What is the water temperature for soap-suds enema?

    E. 99°F
    F. 105°F
    G. 88°F
    H. 115°F

14. The lower plate of a denture is damaged; what is the appropriate action?

    A. Inform the dentist.
    B. Ignore the crack.
    C. Report to the nurse.
    D. Inform the family.

15. Which is incorrect for recording a patient's chart?

    A. Make legible handwriting.
    B. Use a pencil.
    C. Logical writing.
    D. Record what you found and performed.

16. Which is incorrect for an RN assigning you a task?

    A. She should check your qualifications and expertise.
    B. The task should be suitable for you.
    C. Give clear directions.
    D. Delegate all non-RN tasks to you.

17. What is a healthcare agency for a dying patient called?

    A. Hospice
    B. Hospital
    C. Nursing home
    D. Preferred provider organizations

18. What is the proper action for a resident without a bowel movement for five days?

    A. Wait if they use the bathroom tomorrow.
    B. Ask the roommate whether the resident used the bathroom.
    C. Report to the nurse.
    D. Ask the other CNA if the resident used the bathroom that was undocumented.

19.   Which organ does the hepatitis B vaccine protect?

   A. The kidney
   B. The heart
   C. Lungs
   D. The liver

20.   What does nausea signify?

   A. Symptom
   B. Case
   C. Sign
   D. Observation

21.   What is a care plan?

   A. The treatment plan
   B. Flow chart
   C. Nursing care plan
   D. Discharge plan

22.   What are dry hard stools that do not pass called?

   A. Edema
   B. Impaction
   C. Incontinence
   D. Atrophy

23.   What is the standard approach for using the side rails?

   A. Raise them only if the care plan mentions
   B. Raise them at night.
   C. Keep one rail raised.
   D. Raise both sides to make an occupied bed.

24. Wasting or reduced muscle bulk is called?

    A. Disuse
    B. Atelectasis
    C. Withering
    D. Atrophy

25. What is a sitting or semi-sitting position with a raised headend of the bed called?

    A. Sims
    B. Fowler's
    C. Hook's
    D. Lateral

26. What is the loss of ability to express oneself called?

    A. Aphasia
    B. Dysphasia
    C. Dysphagia
    D. Voiceless

27. What is a resident with diabetes more susceptible to?

    A. Infections
    B. Fever
    C. Cancer
    D. Chills

28. Where do you dispose of blood or bodily fluid-contaminated items?

    A. Dirty linen basket
    B. Biohazard box
    C. Dirty utility room
    D. Client room trash can

29. Which personal protective equipment item is best for a CNA managing infectious waste that may splash or spray?

    A. Shoe covers
    B. Mask
    C. Goggles
    D. A face shield

30. What would you do if you forgot to bring the necessary supplies for a procedure?

    A. Tell the client to lie motionless.
    B. Get supplies quickly.
    C. Lower bed and position call light nearby.
    D. Ask the roommate to watch the client while you get your supplies.

31. A client falls and sustains a deep cut. What should you do?

    A. Take them to the emergency.
    B. Help them return to bed.
    C. Wash cut in the bathroom.
    D. Stay with them and call for help.

32. What should you advise a client before taking a 24-hour urine sample?

    A. Bathe before giving a urine sample.
    B. Eat foods without red meat.
    C. Drink 2 L water.
    D. Discard the first voided urine.

33. What should you do if a patient complains of pain during ROM?

    A. Stop.
    B. Continue, ignore the pain.
    C. Do PROM.
    D. Ask the nurse to administer analgesics.

34. Which care principle is the correct teaching for a stroke patient with a weak right arm?

    A. Put his left arm into the shirt first.
    B. Put both arms into the shirt simultaneously.
    C. Put his right arm first.
    D. Choose the arm to go first.

35. Which side should a cane be held?

    A. Strong
    B. Dominant
    C. Weak
    D. Preferred side

36. Which side should you be on to help a patient ambulate after a stroke?

    A. On the patient's weak side.
    B. On the strong side.
    C. Stand behind the patient.
    D. Use a wheelchair.

37. What is a device that replaces body parts called?

    A. Implantation
    B. Pronation
    C. Prognosis
    D. Prosthesis

38. Which statement indicates suicidal ideation?

    A. "We have to go ultimately."
    B. "I don't care what you believe."
    C. "I wish I were dead."
    D. "I need to see a psychiatrist."

39.   Which is the correct approach to a patient's beliefs if they don't belong to your faith?

A. Respect them.
B. Try to change them.
C. Explain how your religion has helped you.
D. Arrange for the patient's clergy to visit him.

40.   Which is not caring for the sexuality of long-term clients?

A. Private time with a partner.
B. Public display of sexuality.
C. Physical appearance.
D. Sexual interactions.

41.   What emotional need should you provide for a resident who cared for her husband until he died recently?

A. Keep her mind busy with other thoughts.
B. Ask her to meet other men.
C. Ask her not to cry.
D. Give her time to grieve.

42.   What is appropriate for a client who wishes to discuss her deceased wife?

A. Call the nurse.
B. Change the topic.
C. Listen and comfort.
D. Ask him to see a counselor.

43.   A terminally ill patient refuses ADLs and throws tantrums, showing which grief stage?

A. Grief
B. Acceptance
C. Anger
D. Denial

44. Which is true for spiritual care?

    A. It needs prescriptions.
    B. Everybody cannot access it.
    C. It connects us with something bigger than us.
    D. It is useless as a therapy.

45. How can you give spiritual care to patients?

    A. Talk to them about your beliefs.
    B. Ask a clergy to visit them.
    C. Do not encourage these topics.
    D. Listen to and respect the client's spiritual concerns.

46. How would you communicate if you are unsure of a gadget's use?

    A. Do not use it.
    B. Seek another way.
    C. Ask the nurse.
    D. Do your best

47. How would you communicate if a resident complains that his children never visit?

    A. Ask others to cheer him up.
    B. Say his children have jobs.
    C. Tell him they will come.
    D. Listen to his feelings.

48. What would you do to find a wet bed when the resident complained someone threw water on their bed?

    A. Scold the resident for urinating in bed.
    B. Change the linen and consider providing frequent bedpans.
    C. Ask the nurse if she would order an indwelling catheter.
    D. Tell the resident to ask for a bedpan when needed.

49. What would you do if a patient says her hearing aids are missing?

   A. Inform the nurse.
   B. Call the family for a replacement.
   C. Tell her to do without them for now.
   D. Tell her to borrow.

50. How should you treat sensitive client information?

   A. Share with other clients.
   B. Keep information confidential.
   C. Share with colleagues in the break room.
   D. Share with the client's relatives.

51. What is the purpose of an incident report?

   A. To find out who is at fault.
   B. To report patient condition.
   C. To record for the family members.
   D. To understand patterns and drift to prevent unwelcoming incidents.

52. Which is not within a patient's right to information?

   A. Wanting to see and discuss one's medical records.
   B. Wanting to see and discuss one's medical bills.
   C. Wanting to know one's procedural side effects.
   D. Wanting to know the roommate's diagnosis from facility staff.

53. You arrive at work to see the charge nurse restraining a patient. What does it mean?

   A. Inform the family.
   B. Avoid the patient so as not to upset them.
   C. Check them 2–hourly for basic needs, circulation, and bathroom requirements.
   D. The nurse will care for them until the restraints are removed.

54.   Which circumstances can raise abetting and aiding charges?

    A. Telling a family member not on the contact list about the patient's diagnosis.
    B. Knowing and not reporting abuse on a patient by a coworker.
    C. Neglecting a patient after a fall.
    D. Abandoning a weak patient in the shower.

55.   Failing to check on a patient's restraints per doctor's orders for patient safety can cause which of these charges?

    A. Incidental harm
    B. Aiding and abetting
    C. Neglect
    D. False documentation

56.   What is the healthcare team's target?

    A. Assigning duties.
    B. Case management.
    C. Give quality care.
    D. Getting reimbursement.

57.   Who is responsible for the nursing team?

    A. A RN
    B. A Supervisor
    C. A case manager
    D. A director of nursing

58.   Who oversees the CNA's work?

    A. A nurse
    B. A doctor
    C. The family
    D. Facility owner

59.   Which is the correct way to address documentation errors?

   A. Draw a single line through it.
   B. Erase it.
   C. Use correction fluid.
   D. Smudge it.

60.   Why is a chain of command necessary for a long-term care facility?

   A. Sustaining communication flow
   B. Creating nursing employment
   C. Ensuring residents adhere to rules
   D. Keeping residents from nurse's station

Time to stop the test; check your answers in Appendix D. Chapter ten is the last practice test of the series.

Answer Key

Q.	1	2	3	4	5	6	7	8	9	10
A.	A	B	A	D	A	C	D	C	A	D

Q.	11	12	13	14	15	16	17	18	19	20
A.	B	A	B	C	D	D	A	A	D	A

Q.	21	22	23	24	25	26	27	28	29	30
A.	C	B	A	D	B	A	A	B	D	C

Q.	31	32	33	34	35	36	37	38	39	40
A.	D	D	A	A	A	A	D	C	A	B

Q.	41	42	43	44	45	46	47	48	49	50
A.	D	C	D	A	D	C	D	B	A	B

Q.	51	52	53	54	55	56	57	58	59	60
A.	D	D	C	B	C	C	D	A	A	A

Answer Explanations

1. A. Clean an incontinent patient quickly. Urine ammonia may damage the skin; bacteria double every 20 minutes in a warm, moist environment.

2. B. Check the water temperature (95°F -105°F) before bathing a client.

3. A. Feces and urine cause skin maceration and irritation, facilitating bacteria proliferation. Clean, dry, and apply a barrier ointment

4. D. Clean and place the dentures into a clean denture cup containing cold water. Label the client's name.

5. A. Always ensure patient privacy, physical or confidential patient information.

6. C. All patients, irrespective of their condition, need oral care.

7. D. A sitz bath soaks a patient or 15 to 20 minutes of water at 100°F up to the hip level after rectal surgery or vaginal births, cleaning and alleviating perineal pain.

8. C. Clean the perineum at the end of a bed bath. Put a cloth beneath the buttocks; wash labia to perineum front-to-back (females); cleanse the penis and scrotum (males). Turn, and clean the buttocks and anal region, and dry.

9. A. Propose care, document rejections, and report it to the charge nurse for the next step.

10. D. CNAs are the first-contact individuals and crucial links between patients and other levels of healthcare.

11. B. Leave all items in the room of a patient in isolation to prevent infection from spreading.

12. A. Making an occupied bed means changing sheets while the patient is on the bed. Cover them with a privacy sheet and elevate the side rail on the

unguarded side. Adjust the bed height per your body mechanics—lower it when finished.

13. B. For soap-suds enema, use lukewarm water at 115°F.

14. C. Cracked dentures can irritate the mouth; report the damage to the nurse.

15. B. Documentation is in permanent ink—correct mistakes according to your facility's policy.

16. D. All non-RN tasks may not be in your job description.

17. A. Hospice care ensures care with dignity and respect without enhancing or shortening life.

18. A. Bowel patterns are unique for everyone, with 3–14 weekly eliminations. Report to the nurse for further investigation or intervention.

19. D. The Hepatitis B vaccine protects the liver.

20. A. Headache, nausea, vomiting, cough, etc., are symptoms of a condition. Signs are physical effects of the disease.

21. C. A care plan starts with patient admission and continues assisting home care.

22. B. The condition of dry, hard stools that choke the rectum is called impaction.

23. A. Raise side rails only if the care plan mentions it.

24. D. Wasting of muscles is called atrophy.

25. B. In high Fowler's, upright posture at 90°, allows chest expansion; the semi-Fowler's position with the headend at 45°–60° helps drainage after surgery.

26. A. A stroke or head injury can damage the brain's speech center, resulting in

aphasia with difficulty in finding appropriate words, understanding speech, and reading and writing problems.

27. A. Uncontrolled diabetes with high blood sugar raises infection possibilities.

28. B. Biohazard box.

29. D. A face shield.

30. C. Lower bed and position call light nearby.

31. D. Stay with injured clients and call for help.

32. D. Discard first voided urine.

33. A. Stop ROM if a patient complains of pain and reports.

34. A. Teach the resident to dress the affected side with the unaffected side first. While undressing, he should take out the unaffected side first.

35. A. Using a cane on the stronger side automatically shifts the body weight to that side.

36. A. Stand on the weak side of the patient for support.

37. D. A prosthesis is a device that replaces accidentally or surgically missing body parts.

38. C. Patients with suicidal ideation often talk about death.

39. A. Respect the client's beliefs.

40. B. Sexuality does not mean public display of sexual acts.

41. D. Give time to grieve her spouse.

42. C. Listen and try to give comfort.

43. D. Anger, Kübler-Ross's second stage of grief.

44. A. Spiritual care connects us with something bigger than us, rebuilds our faith and trust, and calms our minds.

45. D. Listen to and respect clients' spiritual concerns and beliefs to care for their spiritual needs.

46. C. Communication should be flowing, direct, and genuine for best serving the patient.

47. D. Sometimes, empathic listening does all the talking.

48. B. Change the linen and consider providing frequent bedpans instead of embarrassing or blaming them. Try to ascertain the reason behind a behavior.

49. A. Contacting the family is outside your job description. Perform the following for a missing object:

    i.   Search thoroughly.
    ii.   Inform the nurse.
    iii. Fill up the requisite forms.

50. B. Patient information is confidential.

51. D. Incident reports help understand patterns and drift to prevent the recurrence of unwelcoming incidents.

52. D. HIPAA prevents access to others' medical information unless explicitly permitted.

53. C. Perform your assignments on the patient as best as possible. Check the restraints for safety.

54. B. Knowing and not reporting abuse on a patient by a coworker is a legal crime called abetting and aiding.

55. C. Neglect is carelessness and failure to provide adequate patient care.

56. C. The healthcare team acknowledges that no one has all the knowledge for patient care. Team management ensures quality care by obtaining input from specific care segments.

57. D. The director of nursing (DON) manages nursing staff, budgets, and patients and families.

58. A. A registered nurse (RN) or licensed practical or vocational nurse (LPN/LVN) supervises a nursing assistant daily.

59. A. Charting mistake correction rules are:

    i.   Never conceal the mistake.
    ii.   Draw a single line across the error to show the entry.
    iii. Add your initials and date.
    iv.   Write correct information.

60. A. To ensure open and productive communication.

Chapter Ten: Practice Test 5

Let us begin with practice test 5. Remember, practice tests are just that; the questions are close approximates of what you may expect in the actual test. Go through the test patterns, the question types, and the answers the test-takers want, but do not memorize the questions.

1.   What is crucial to recognize in a patient who wants to shower once weekly?

   A. Educating patients on the facility's shower policy
   B. Acknowledging patients' cultural needs
   C. Risks for impending depression
   D. Notifying the family about hygiene issues

2.   What is not the risk of inadequate water drinking?

   A. Swollen gum
   B. Skin infection
   C. Mouth sores
   D. Bad breath

3.   Which of these is not an indication of pain in an 85-year-old?

   A. Insomnia
   B. Isolation
   C. Agitation
   D. Social participation

4.   Which is not the aim of giving ADLs?

A. Comfort
B. Security
C. Dissuade self-care
D. Safety

5.   A client is independent but slow. What should be your attitude toward giving ADLs?

A. Remain ready to help when needed.
B. Ask her to let you help for faster task completion.
C. Ask her to take baths on opposite shifts.
D. Ask her politely to be a little quicker because others need your assistance.

6.   Which part of the body would you rather avoid applying lotion?

A. Fingers
B. Arms
C. Feet
D. Toes

7.   Which is accurate for shaving?

A. Use long upward strokes.
B. Rinse the blade after three strokes.
C. Shave upwards on the neck.
D. Use upward strokes for the chin.

8.   Which of these must be considered while giving hair care?

A. Ethnicity
B. Mobility
C. Hygiene
D. Age

9.   What does ADL represent?

A. Assisted Daily Living
B. Activities of Daily Living
C. Assist Disabled Living
D. Activities that Drive Life

10.   What is the best way to keep a facility free of foul odor?

A. Open all windows
B. Regular use of air freshener
C. Timely emptying of bedpans and changing linens
D. Hospitals smell bad

11.   What is decubitus ulcer also called?

A. Perforation
B. Ulcerated cyst
C. Ulcerated tumor
D. Pressure sores.

12.   Which is not used for contractures?

A. Bandaging
B. Physical therapy
C. Hand roll
D. Frequent repositioning

13.   A resident with 90/60 BP is feeling faint. What is the diagnosis?

A. Hypothermia
B. Hypotension
C. Hypoglycemia
D. Hypertension

14. Which is best to diminish swelling?

    A. Cold compression
    B. Moist bandage
    C. Hot compress
    D. Dry bandage pressure

15. How not to communicate with dysphasic (difficulty speaking) patients?

    A. Use visual aids.
    B. Encourage sense organ usage to convey.
    C. Finish their words.
    D. Complement their efforts.

16. Which is the most likely method to prevent residents from self-inflicted harm?

    A. Isolation
    B. Additional staff
    C. Restraints
    D. Observation schedule 24/7

17. What is not a Heimlich maneuver?

    A. Do immediately if a resident is coughing.
    B. You can do it on yourself.
    C. Use a fist.
    D. Your hand must be around the xiphoid and the umbilicus.

18. What is avoided for measuring BP?

    A. The resident's feet are on the floor.
    B. The resident lies with feet elevated.
    C. BP is slightly higher in the AM.
    D. The resident must not talk.

19. What is the medical term for passing gas?

   A. Fascia
   B. Fibula
   C. Flatus
   D. Wind

20. Which is inaccurate while donning gloves?

   A. Latex gloves are best.
   B. Handwash before and after wearing gloves.
   C. Avoid touching the glove's outer surface during removal.
   D. Peel the glove away from you with the inner surface coming out.

21. Why are axillary temperatures lower than other forms of temperature taking?

   A. It is a deeper area.
   B. It is at the back.
   C. It is briefly recorded.
   D. It is outside the body.

22. What is the normal pulse rate for children?

   A. 60–100 beats/minute
   B. 80–130 beats/minute
   C. 70–120 beats/minute
   D. 50–80 beats/minute

23. What is the correct handwashing procedure?

   A. Friction for 15 seconds
   B. Antibacterial soap only
   C. Longer friction time for soaps that do not produce lather
   D. Turning off the tap with a paper towel

24. Which doesn't signify impending death?

    A. Unstable BP
    B. Cool extremities
    C. Wanting to eat
    D. Labored breathing

25. Why is oral temperature taking popular?

    A. Most accurate.
    B. Most cost-beneficial.
    C. Residents accept only this method.
    D. Least inconvenient.

26. What is the most convenient choice for a resident ordered to drink two-hourly 240cc of fluids?

    A. A 5 oz can of juice
    B. A 8 oz can of juice
    C. A 3 oz can of juice
    D. A 7 oz can of juice

27. Which of these is CNAs' task concerning IV fluids?

    A. Watch the IV line and report.
    B. Not your responsibility.
    C. Prepare the solution.
    D. Start the IV line.

28. What is the best method for recording temperatures in infants?

    A. Oral
    B. Rectal
    C. Temporal
    D. Axillary

29.   What is the correct depth for CPR compression?

    A. 2"
    B. 2.5"
    C. 1"
    D. 1.5"

30.   During CPR, what is the rate of providing breaths to a patient?

    A. One breath every 4 seconds
    B. One breath every 5 seconds
    C. One breath every 6 seconds
    D. One breath every 7 seconds

31.   You had a busy schedule and could only empty the Foley bag at the end of your 12-hour shift. Which of the urine output is a concern?

    A. 1,000 mL
    B. 350 mL
    C. 500 mL
    D. 1800 mL

32.   The diet of a strict dysphasia patient should not have which of these items?

    A. Apple sauce
    B. Jello
    C. Mashed potato
    D. Regular orange juice.

33.   Which is a PROM?

    A. Hold the arm and gently perform a range of movements.
    B. You move your arm.
    C. Ask the resident to move the arm.
    D. Use resistance exercise.

34. Which muscles are most injury-prone?

    A. Arm
    B. Leg
    C. Neck
    D. Back

35. What is best to encourage resident's independence?

    A. Allow the resident to soil their beds to motivate them to use toilets.
    B. Roommates should help with chores.
    C. Allow the resident to participate in morning care.
    D. Provide necessary items for self-care and leave the room.

36. What is not an assisting device's purpose?

    A. Dressing
    B. Eating
    C. Ambulating
    D. Restraint

37. Which therapy describes restorative nursing?

    A. Occupational nursing
    B. Restorative nursing
    C. Therapeutic nursing
    D. Proactive nursing

38. When is the normal aging process best represented?

    A. Declining body and mental faculties.
    B. People grow dependent and childlike.
    C. 65 years old.
    D. Beginning of dementia.

39. What is an appropriate approach for an excessively demanding resident?

    A. Do her routines in your available time rather than when she wishes.

B. Avoid her room after finishing her tasks.

C. Tell her others are more in need of you.

D. Ask if you performed all her needs before leaving her room.

40.   Who should you report if a resident avoids specific food for religious reasons?

A. Dietitian

B. Charge nurse

C. Family

D. Doctor

41.   What action can meet a male resident's social needs?

A. Compliment him for accomplishing new things.

B. Keep his room clean and tidy.

C. Use postural support as necessary.

D. Serve hot meals timely.

42.   What step is followed for a confused client?

A. Keep him isolated.

B. Ignore him until he makes sense.

C. Restrain him.

D. Help him recognize known things and people.

43.   How can you provide a sense of security?

A. Closing the door

B. Explaining procedures

C. Using Restraints

D. Playing a television series during ADLs

44.   Why must you close the door and curtain to give postmortem care?

A. No one should see the resident.

B. Always maintain respect and dignity.

C. Close the curtain only.
D. Closing doors and curtains is unnecessary.

45. What is the best way to relieve stress?

A. Mindful meditation
B. Reading
C. Gossiping about residents
D. Eating

46. Which is not good for conflict resolution?

A. Own your mistakes and apologize.
B. Emotional decision-making.
C. Organize meetings for resolution.
D. Positive attitude.

47. What is a proper "register" in communication?

A. Facility-supported client record
B. A list of medical terminology
C. Method to help clients recall
D. Ways of communication

48. What is the significance of touch as communication?

A. Naturally used
B. Culture-specific
C. Shows authority
D. Used in direct caregiving

49. What is best while asking questions?

A. Avoid stacking questions.
B. Voice your opinion.
C. Ask difficult questions first.
D. Use a yes–no format.

50.   What does a resident receive on admission to a long-term care facility?

    A. Informed consent
    B. A copy of the resident's Bill of Rights
    C. Activity schedules
    D. Facility menu card

51.   Who handles residents' finances?

    A. The resident
    B. Supervisors
    C. Family
    D. Lawyer

52.   Who should you not share resident information with?

    A. Charge nurse
    B. Doctor
    C. Best friend on a weekly visit
    D. Physical therapist

53.   Which is violating privacy rights?

    A. The nurse discussed the patient's condition with the next shift's coworker.
    B. Two CNAs discuss a patient over lunch.
    C. A CNA talks about a patient to an EMT Who will transfer the patient.
    D. A CNA and a nurse discuss the care plan with the patient.

54.   Which is not included in the Patient's Bill of Rights?

    A. Right to terminate their lives.
    B. Right to obtain privacy and respect.
    C. Right to know about their medical condition.
    D. Right to wear their clothes.

55. What should you do if you notice a CNA neglecting their duty?

    A. Ignore.
    B. Do their task.
    C. Complaining to other coworkers.
    D. Report to the nurse.

56. Which is not the domain of the CNA profession?

    A. Teamwork
    B. Enthusiastic approach
    C. Isolated work
    D. Communicative approach

57. What information is vital before transferring a client?

    A. Patient's medical diagnosis
    B. Patient's name and room number
    C. Spouse's name
    D. Room phone number

58. Facility guidelines on CNA duty have all except?

    A. Follow a dress code.
    B. Discounting professional training.
    C. Report to a charge nurse.
    D. Report on time.

59. What best defines a CNA role?

    A. Licensed to prescribe diet
    B. Transcribes doctor's orders
    C. A graduate nurse licensed to practice nursing
    D. Certified to assist registered practice nurses

60. Which behavior is shown by a CNA who accepts a new assignment from the charge nurse without complaint?

A. Flexibility
B. Consideration
C. Responsibility
D. Curiosity

Answer Key

Q.	1	2	3	4	5	6	7	8	9	10
A.	B	A	D	C	A	D	C	A	B	B

Q.	11	12	13	14	15	16	17	18	19	20
A.	D	A	B	A	B	C	A	B	C	A

Q.	21	22	23	24	25	26	27	28	29	30
A.	D	C	D	C	D	B	A	B	A	C

Q.	31	32	33	34	35	36	37	38	39	40
A.	B	D	A	D	C	D	B	A	D	B

Q.	41	42	43	44	45	46	47	48	49	50
A.	A	D	B	B	A	B	D	B	A	B

Q.	51	52	53	54	55	56	57	58	59	60
A.	A	C	B	A	D	C	B	B	D	A

Answer Explanations

1. B. Nurses' concept of "dirty" may not tally with patients' cultural needs for self-care routines that should be accepted unless there are other reasons for daily washing.

2. A. Inadequate oral fluids can cause dehydration, predisposing to skin breakdown and infection, bad breath, and mouth sores.

3. D. An elderly person refusing to participate socially strongly indicates pain.

4. C. Person-centered therapy always aims for independence and self-sufficiency. While ADLs provide safety, security, and comfort, patients are encouraged to participate as much as possible.

5. A. Response time slows down with aging. Still, patients' independence should always be valued.

6. D. Wet and moist toes can attract skin maceration and fungal and bacterial growth.

7. C. Wet the skin and shave with short strokes, following the direction of hair growth. Rinse after every stroke.

8. A. Hair care vastly varies between ethnicity and culture.

9. B. ADL denotes Activities of Daily Living, CNAs' responsibility.

10. B. A pleasing setting promotes health. Dispose of or clean used items promptly and correctly.

11. D. Pressure sores are more appropriate due to constant contact with body surfaces in immobile patients.

12. A. Contractures follow joint stiffening and degeneration; bandaging can aggravate this.

13. B. Hypotension is BP < 90/60, with symptoms like dizziness.

14. A. Heat packs are for backache, moist bandages are for burns, dry bandage pressure stops bleeding, and cold packs are for reducing swelling.

15. B. Dysphasia may follow neurological or local problems like surgery for oral cavity tumors. Patients cannot talk but are aware. Do not finish their words yourself.

16. C. Order restraints for patients that can harm themselves.

17. A. A coughing resident can dislodge food in the respiratory tract, not needing the Heimlich maneuver.

18. B. Avoid taking BP in a supine patient with elevated legs.

19. C. The medical term for passing gas or burping is flatus.

20. A. Latex gloves can cause allergies.

21. D. Axillary regions are outside the body and record lower temperatures than other methods.

22. C. Children have pulse rates of 70–120 beats/minute; one-year-olds can have higher.

23. D. Turn off the tap with a paper towel after hand wash.

24. C. Lowered appetite indicates the body's shutdown.

25. D. Due to its access, oral temperature taking is popular.

26. B. One oz is 30 cc; an eight oz can is 240cc

27. A. CNAs should watch the IV and report any issues to the nurse.

28. C. Rectal temperature reflects core body temperature. Axilla is unsuitable because of its looseness.

29. A. Compress at least 2" of the chest to perfuse the brain. Pressure >2.4" is not recommended.

30. C. The correct rate for providing breaths during CPR is 1 breath every 6 seconds, or 10 breaths/minute.

31. B. Urine output should be at least 30 mL/minute. 350 mL/12 hours is a concern and can mean acute kidney shutdown.

32. D. A dysphagia (swallowing problems) diet should include thickened juice rather than a regular one.

33. A. PROM is doing a passive range of movements you execute for the resident.

34. D. Back muscles are the most injury-prone.

35. C. Allow the resident to work independently and assist when necessary.

36. D. Assisting devices like canes help residents with task performance. Restraints undermine it.

37. B. You cannot create a rehabilitation plan but assist.

38. A. Medical history, lifestyle, and genetics affect aging, beginning after age 30—vision, hearing, and organ function decline. Muscle loss affects strength and flexibility: physical activity, proper food, and socialization slow aging.

39. D. Show your care and concern for the client, who can be anxious or lonely.

40. B. Report to the nurse. Reasons for special diets are religion, medical conditions, and food allergies.

41. A. Social rewards include praise and attention.

42. D. Spending time with the client examining familiar objects and people helps them to reorient and relax.

43. B. Doing something unexpected or rushing a client causes anxiety and fear.

44. B. Provide patient dignity and respect after death.

45. A. Mindful meditation can provide spiritual connection.

46. B. Emotional decisions are often impulsive and miss the bigger picture.

47. D. Situations determine conversational formality. Work registration uses unique terms like NPO and DNR. Registers are common to all languages, and we know when to speak formally and casually.

48. B. Touch is a vital communication tool. However, certain cultures restrict touching, particularly by the opposing gender.

49. A. While you can learn more from clients by asking about their health and building relationships, avoid too many questions at a time.

50. B. Nursing homes and long-term care establishments provide new residents with a language-friendly Residents Bill of Rights, assuring respectful treatment.

51. A. Residents have the right to handle their finances or choose someone for it.

52. C. Only those directly involved with care can share information.

53. B. CNAs informally discussing a patient could violate patient privacy.

54. A. The Bill of Rights does not provide for patients' right to end life.

55. D. Report any negligence to the nurse.

56. C. CNA work is collaborative and communicative, but CNAs should finish their assignments.

57. B. Obtain patients' names and room numbers before transferring patients.

58. B. CNA training is a prerequisite to employment.

59. D. CNAs are certified to work under the charge nurse's supervision.

60. A. A flexible nursing assistant accepts a new task readily.

Conclusion

A challenging and competitive examination like the CNA test needs a good guidebook. As an educator, I know the anxiety of examination preparation, which entails collecting the best study material, following the best study methods, and keeping examination fears at bay. All these elements can derail the prospects of even a first-class student.

You aim to be a nursing assistant because your career goals are serious, and you are passionate about this profession. Being a CNA will give you practical experience and theoretical knowledge. It can widen the scope for bettering your career.

To that goal, my book on the CNA test offered the best and most exhaustive guidelines on theory and practicum. The book aims to help you gain knowledge and confidence. Leaving a good review on the Amazon platform will enable other aspirants to seek it.

References

American Red Cross. 2013. "Third Edition Nurse Assistant Training." https://qualitycnatraining.com/wp-content/uploads/2020/04/CNA-Textbook.pdf.

Ana Gascon Ivey. 2021. "What Is the Patient's Bill of Rights?" GoodRx. GoodRx. August 19, 2021. https://www.goodrx.com/insurance/health-insurance/patients-bill-of-rights#:~:text=The%20goal%20was%20to%20protect.

"CNA Certification Requirement by State || RegisteredNursing.org." 2023. Www.registerednursing.org. June 22, 2023. https://www.registerednursing.org/certified-nursing-assistant/certification/.

"Continuity of Care: NCLEX-RN || RegisteredNursing.org." 2023. Registered Nursing. October 11, 2023. https://www.registerednursing.org/nclex/continuity-care/.

"Emergency Response for CNA and HHA." 2022. Ceufast.com. August 18, 2022. https://ceufast.com/course/emergency-response-for-cna-and-hha.

Hilgers, Laura . 2023. "How One Healthcare System Is Addressing a Talent Shortage | LinkedIn." Www.linkedin.com. February 7, 2023. https://www.linkedin.com/business/talent/blog/learning-and-development/how-one-healthcare-system-is-addressing-a-talent-shortage.

Kelly, M. 1989. "The Omnibus Budget Reconciliation Act of 1987. A Policy Analysis." The Nursing Clinics of North America 24 (3): 791–94. https://pubmed.ncbi.nlm.nih.gov/2671955/.

McLeod, Saul. 2018. "Maslow's Hierarchy of Needs." Canada College. Simply Psychology. https://canadacollege.edu/dreamers/docs/Maslows-Hierarchy-of-Needs.pdf.

Mcleod, Saul. 2023. "Erik Erikson's Stages of Psychosocial Development." Simply Psychology. Simply Scholar. October 16, 2023. https://www.simplypsychology.org/Erik-Erikson.html.

Population Reference Bureau. 2023. "Fact Sheet: U.S. Dementia Trends." PRB. 2023. https://www.prb.org/resources/fact-sheet-u-s-dementia-trends/.

Prometric. n.d. "Generic Nurse Aide Clinical Skills Checklist." Https://Www.prometric.com/Sites/Default/Files/FL_CNA_ClinicalSkillsChecklist.pdf.

"Recording Care through the PACE Framework." 2020. Health Research Authority. April 1, 2020. https://www.hra.nhs.uk/planning-and-improving-research/application-summaries/research-summaries/recording-care-through-the-pace-framework/#:~:text=The%20PACE%20documentation%20was%20also.

Sandquist Reuter, Myra . 2022. "2.2 Ethical and Legal Responsibilities of the Nursing Assistant." Wtcs.pressbooks.pub. https://wtcs.pressbooks.pub/nurseassist/chapter/2-2-ethical-and-legal-responsibilities-of-the-nursing-assistant/#:~:text=Ethical%20Responsibilities%20of%20the%20Nursing.

Shmerling, Robert. 2015. "First, Do No Harm - Harvard Health Blog." Harvard Health Blog. October 14, 2015. https://www.health.harvard.edu/blog/first-do-no-harm-201510138421.

sprinto. 2023. "What Is HIPAA Compliance? [2024 Updated Guide]." Sprinto. September 15, 2023. https://sprinto.com/blog/

hipaa-compliance/#:~:text=The%20Health%20Insurance%20Portability%20 and.

Suzanne Ball, Winona . 2021. "CNA Skills Test: Your 5-Step Success Plan [Incl. 19 Videos]." CNA Practice Tests. September 4, 2021. https://cna.plus/pass-cna-skills-test-how-to/.

Teoli, Dac, and Sassan Ghassemzadeh. 2020. "Patient Self-Determination Act." PubMed. Treasure Island (FL): StatPearls Publishing. 2020. https://www.ncbi.nlm.nih.gov/books/NBK538297/.

Toney-Butler, Tammy J., and Jennifer M. Thayer. 2023. "Nursing Process." PubMed. Treasure Island (FL): StatPearls Publishing. April 10, 2023. https://www.ncbi.nlm.nih.gov/books/NBK499937/#:~:text=The%20nursing%20 process%20functions%20as.

U.S. Bureau of Labor Statistics. 2019. "Nursing Assistants and Orderlies : Occupational Outlook Handbook: : U.S. Bureau of Labor Statistics." Bls.gov. September 4, 2019. https://www.bls.gov/ooh/healthcare/nursing-assistants.htm.

Whitenton, Linda, and Marty Walker. 2009. CNA Certified Nursing Assistant Exam Cram. Pearson Education.

Made in the USA
Columbia, SC
29 December 2023

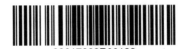

29617662R00122